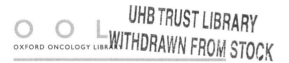

Systemic Treatment of Non-Small-Cell Lung Cancer

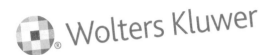

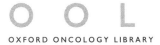

OXFORD ONCOLOGY LIBRARY

Systemic Treatment of Non-Small-Cell Lung Cancer

Edited by

Giuseppe Giaccone

Chief of the Medical Oncology Branch,
National Cancer Institute (NCI) of the
National Institutes of Health (NIH),
Bethesda, Maryland, USA

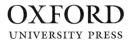

OXFORD

UNIVERSITY PRESS

OXFORD

UNIVERSITY PRESS

Great Clarendon Street, Oxford OX2 6DP
United Kingdom

Oxford University Press is a department of the University of Oxford.
It furthers the University's objective of excellence in research, scholarship,
and education by publishing worldwide. Oxford is a registered trade mark of
Oxford University Press in the UK and in certain other countries

First published in 2012
Impression: 1

British Library Cataloguing in Publication Data
Data available

Library of Congress Cataloging in Publication Data
Data available

ISBN 978-0-19-958048-4

Printed in Great Britain
Clays Ltd, St Ives plc

Contents

Abbreviations

ACCP	American College of Chest Physicians
AJCC	American Joint Committee on Cancer
ALK	anaplastic lymphoma kinase
ALPI	Adjuvant Lung Project Italy
ANITA	Adjuvant Navelbine International Trialist Association
BAC	bronchioloalveolar carcinoma
CALGB	Cancer and Leukemia Group B
CCS	cancer cachexia syndrome
CDK	cyclin-dependent kinase
CISCA	cisplatin vs carboplatin meta-analysis
COPD	chronic obstructive pulmonary disease
CT	computed tomography
cTNM	clinical staging
3-DCRT	3D conformal radiotherapy
DSMC	Data Safety Monitoring Committee
EBUS-TBNA	endobronchial ultrasound with transbronchial needle aspiration
ECOG	Eastern Cooperative Oncology Group
EGFR	epidermal growth factor receptor
EUS-FNA	endoscopic ultrasound with fine needle-aspiration
GC	gemcitabine/cisplatin
HDAC	histone deacetylase inhibitors
HPV	human papilloma virus
HR	hazard ratio
IALT	International Adjuvant Lung Trial
IASLC	International Association for the Study of Lung Cancer
IFCT	Intergroupe Francophone de Cancérologie Thoracique
IGF	insulin-like growth factor
IGFR	insulin growth factor receptor
IGRT	image-guided radiation therapy

IMRT	intensity modulated radiation therapy
IPD	individual data based
ITC	isolated tumour cells
kV	kilovoltage
LACE	Lung Adjuvant Cisplatin Evaluation
LANSCLC	locally advanced NSCLC
LOH	loss of heterozygosity
MAP	mitogen activated protein
MEK	mitogen-activated protein kinase
MRI	magnetic resonance imaging
mTOR	mammalian target of rapamycin
MV	megavoltage
nAChR	nicotinic acetylcholine receptor subunits
NCIC-CTG	National Institute of Canada Clinical Trials Group
NSCLC	non-small-cell lung cancer
PC	paclitaxel/carboplatin
PET	positron emission tomography
PFS	progression free survival
PO	post-operative
PS	performance status
pTNM	pathological staging
RADIANT	Randomized Double-blind Trial in Adjuvant NSCLC with Tarceva
RB	retinoblastoma
RT	radiotherapy
SCLC	small-cell lung cancer
SNP	single nucleotide polymorphisms
TKI	tyrosine kinase inhibitors
TNM	tumour node metastasis
TRAIL	tumour necrosis factor-related apoptosis-inducing ligand
TS	thymidylate synthase
TSG	tumour suppressor genes
UFT	uracil plus tegafur

UTR	untranslated region
VALSG	Veterans' Affairs Lung Study Group
VAS	visual analogue scale
VATS	video assisted thoracotomy
VEGF	vascular endothelial growth factor
WHO	World Health Organization

Contributors

Paul Baas
Netherlands Cancer Institute,
Amsterdam, Netherlands

Benjamin Besse
Department of Medicine,
Institut Gustave Roussy,
Villejuif, France

Hak Choy
Radiation Oncology, Moncrief
Building, Dallas, TX, USA

Sofie De Craene
Department of Respiratory
Medicine & Thoracic
Oncology, University
Hospital, Ghent, Belgium

Margaret Edwards
Radiation Oncology, Moncrief
Building, Dallas, TX, USA

Adi F. Gazdar
Hamon Center for
Therapeutic Oncology
Research, Simmons Cancer
Center, University of Texas
Southwestern Medical
Center, Dallas, TX ,USA

Giuseppe Giaccone
Chief of the Medical
Oncology Branch,
National Cancer Institute
(NCI) of the National
Institutes of Health (NIH),
Bethesda, Maryland, USA

Pasi A. Jänne
Dana-Farber Cancer Institute,
Boston, MA , USA

Jill E. Larsen
Hamon Center for
Therapeutic Oncology
Research, Simmons Cancer
Center, University of Texas
Southwestern Medical
Center, Dallas, TX, USA

John D. Minna
Hamon Center for
Therapeutic Oncology
Research, Simmons Cancer
Center, University of Texas
Southwestern Medical
Center, Dallas, TX, USA

Taylor M. Ortiz
Dana-Farber Cancer Institute,
Boston, MA, USA

Arun Rajan
Medical Oncology Branch,
National Cancer Institute,
Bethesda, MD

Frances A. Shepherd
Princess Margaret Hospital,
University Health Network,
University of Toronto,
Toronto, Ontario, Canada

Jean-Charles Soria
Department of Medicine,
Institut Gustave Roussy,
Villejuif, France

Kurt G. Tournoy
Department of Respiratory
Medicine & Thoracic
Oncology, University
Hospital; Lung
Oncological Network Ghent
(LONG), Ghent, Belgium

Wilma Uyterlinde
Netherlands Cancer Institute,
Amsterdam, Netherlands

Jan P. van Meerbeeck
Department of Respiratory
Medicine & Thoracic
Oncology, University Hospital;
Lung Oncological Network
Ghent (LONG), Ghent,
Belgium

Paul Wheatley-Price
Ottawa Hospital Cancer
Centre, University of Ottawa,
Ottawa, Ontario, Canada

Chapter 1

Molecular biology of lung cancer for the clinician

Adi F. Gazdar, Jill E. Larsen, and John D. Minna

Key points

- The molecular biology of lung cancer is highly complex with numerous genetic, epigenetic, and cytological changes present in all lung cancers
- Considerable progress has been made in identifying the key 'driver' mutations essential for the appearance or maintenance of the cancer phenotype
- The molecular changes characterizing the major forms of lung cancer, small-cell, adenocarcinoma, and squamous cell carcinomas are distinct
- Lung cancer arising in lifetime non smokers (mainly adenocarcinomas) constitute a distinct entity
- Advances in medicine and the selection of cases for individualized medicine require greater accuracy in histological classification of non-small-cell lung cancers
- Global approaches to studying the complex lung cancer genome landscape have identified many actual or potential targets for therapy
- Translation of our considerable laboratory knowledge of lung cancer biology to the clinic will enable us to achieve the goal of personalized medicine for all or most lung cancer patients in the not too distant future.

1.1 Introduction

Lung cancer is the leading cause of cancer deaths in the world. Recent advances in diagnosis, therapy, and management have made only modest improvements in overall survival. These grim facts have resulted in a growing enthusiasm for individualized medicine based on identification of targets in individual tumours. Technological advances in global techniques for interrogating the cancer genome and its landscape have resulted in huge strides in our knowledge and understanding of lung cancer pathogenesis. This enormous body of theoretical knowledge is slowly being translated into clinical care.

Lung cancer, as with most solid tumours, is remarkably complex and each individual tumour contains numerous genetic, epigenetic, and cytological changes. One important question is how we can distinguish the modest number of 'driver' mutations, essential for the appearance or maintenance of the cancer cell phenotype from the much more numerous 'passenger' mutations which make little or no contribution to the cancer cell. Solid tumours do not arise *de novo*, but only after a series of sequential preneoplastic changes that occur over many years or decades. Until recently, the clinic-pathological classification of lung cancer into small-cell (SCLC, representing 15–20%) and non-small-cell (NSCLC, representing 80–85% of cases) categories was sufficient for most purposes. However, the use of therapies that target specific subtypes of NSCLC has made histological distinction important, especially between adenocarcinomas and squamous cell carcinomas. The two main disease categories of lung cancer are generally classified based on differences in histological, clinical, and neuroendocrine characteristics. NSCLC and SCLC also differ molecularly with many genetic alterations exhibiting subtype specificity. Additionally, molecular studies of NSCLC have revealed considerable differences between the subtypes of NSCLC, particularly the two most common subtypes: adenocarcinoma and squamous cell carcinoma.

Another important point is that the lung is not a single anatomic structure, but consists of central (conducting) and peripheral (gaseous exchange) compartments. Squamous cell carcinomas and SCLC mainly arise in the central compartment, while adenocarcinomas are usually peripherally arising tumours.

1.2 The hallmarks of lung cancer

Hanahan and Weinberg described the 'hallmarks of cancer' as six essential alterations in cell physiology that collectively dictate malignant growth. These acquired capabilities are described in Table 1.1, along with examples for each hallmark. Acquisition of the hallmarks results in acquisition of an enabling characteristic, namely genomic instability, a characteristic feature of malignant transformation. Genomic instability can manifest itself at the chromosomal level (with loss or gain of genomic material, translocations, and microsatellite instability), at the nucleotide level (with single or several nucleotide base changes), or in the transcriptome (with altered gene expression). Abnormalities are typically targeted to proto-oncogenes, tumour suppressor genes (TSGs), DNA repair genes, and other genes that can promote outgrowth of affected cells. The acquisition of the hallmarks and subsequently of genomic instability permit the cancer genome to develop the numerous driver and passenger mutations characteristic of solid cancers.

1.3 The multistage pathogenesis of lung cancers

Transformation from a normal to malignant lung cancer phenotype is thought to arise in a multi-step fashion, through a series of genetic and epigenetic alterations, ultimately evolving into invasive cancer by clonal expansion. These changes precede the onset of histologically identifiable preneoplastic lesions. Each of the major types of lung cancer follows its own distinct pathway. The best defined pathway is for squamous cell carcinoma as the sequential events can be followed by endoscopy. As there are no squamous cells normally present in the respiratory epithelium, these cancers arise from squamous metaplastic changes in the central airways. Progressively severe dysplastic changes follow, with the development of squamous carcinoma in situ and finally invasive cancer. The changes in the peripheral compartment cannot be followed by sequential sampling, and are less well defined. A lesion known as atypical adenomatous hyperplasia is believed to be the preneoplastic precursor for peripheral adenocarcinomas, followed by non-invasive bronchioloalveolar carcinoma (BAC) and then by invasive adenocarcinomas. Unfortunately the term BAC has been used inconsistently, with some pathologists using it for tumours with a large BAC component and small invasive component. This practice has led to considerable confusion, and it has recently been proposed that the term BAC be abandoned in favour of pulmonary adenocarcinoma in situ. The changes preceding small-cell lung cancer are not well defined, but extensive molecular changes in the respiratory epithelium precede its development, indicating that widespread and extensive damage may predispose to this carcinoma.

Multiple molecular changes, characteristic of those present in invasive cancers, can be found in the respiratory epithelium of smokers, more so in the central compartment than in the periphery. These field effects predispose to lung cancer and the changes progressively increase during multistage pathogenesis.

The identification and characterization of these molecular changes in lung cancer is of fundamental importance for improving the prevention, early detection, treatment and palliation of this disease. The overall goal is to translate these findings to the clinic by using molecular alterations as: 1) biomarkers for early detection; 2) targets for prevention; 3) tools for new molecular approaches; 4) signatures for personalizing prognosis and therapy selection for each patient; and 5) targets to specifically kill or inhibit the growth of lung cancer in patients.

The two main disease categories of lung cancer, NSCLC (representing 80–85% of cases) and SCLC (representing 15–20%) are generally classified based on differences in histological, clinical and neuroendocrine characteristics. NSCLC and SCLC can also differ molecularly with many genetic alterations exhibiting subtype specificity. Additionally, molecular studies of NSCLC have also revealed considerable differences between the subtypes of NSCLC, particularly the two most common subtypes: adenocarcinoma and squamous cell carcinoma.

1.3.1 Epidemiology, susceptibility and smoke exposure in lung cancer

Eighty-five per cent of lung cancers are caused by tobacco smoke where exposure to carcinogens present in tobacco smoke leads to the acquisition of genetic mutations that may eventually initiate carcinogenesis. However, not all lung cancers arise in smokers, and not all smokers will develop lung cancer. Thus, inherited factors must be involved which predispose an individual to developing lung cancer—either by increasing susceptibility to the damaging effects of carcinogen exposure, or by increasing susceptibility regardless of smoking history. Worldwide, approximately 25% of lung cancer cases are not attributable to smoking. These cases occur more frequently in women, especially in Asian countries, target the distal airways, and are commonly adenocarcinomas. Coupled with molecular data that indicates strikingly different mutation patterns between known lung cancer genes such as *KRAS*, *EGFR*, and *TP53* and clinical data in relation to response to targeted therapies—it has now been suggested that lung cancer in never smokers be considered a distinct disease from the more common tobacco smoke-related lung cancer.

Many studies have examined the effect of single nucleotide polymorphisms (SNPs) on the risk of developing lung cancer. The reported risk effect in these studies is generally modest and often inconsistent, explaining why none are in routine use. However, meta-analyses as well as use of whole-genome SNP microarrays may hold the key to identifying robust and possible synergistic interactions between the modest affect of multiple SNPs. Of note, lung cancer risk was recently associated with genomic variation at 15q24/q25.1 by three separate studies simultaneously that used whole-genome SNP microarrays. While the conclusions of the three studies differed in whether the risk is conferred directly with cancer or through nicotine addiction, the genes within this locus—which include several genes encoding nicotinic acetylcholine receptor subunits (nAChR)—represent important targets for further functional analyses.

1.4 **Major driver mutations for lung cancer**

Many oncogenes and TSGs have been identified by the mapping of copy-number changes throughout the cancer genome. This process has been greatly aided by the widespread use of high resolution microarray analyses that narrow in on these aberrant regions to detect focal amplifications and deletions often spanning only a handful of genes.

Oncogenic activation typically occurs by gene amplification, point mutation, rearrangement, or through gene over-expression by other mechanisms including those mediated by microRNAs. These changes can result in persistent upregulation of mitogenic growth signals which induce cell growth. While promoting the malignant transformation of a cell, persistent upregulation of a particular growth signal or pathway can also result in 'oncogenic addiction'—whereby the cell becomes dependent upon the aberrant oncogenic signaling for survival. Oncogene addiction presents an obvious target for therapeutics; remove or inhibit the oncogenic signal and an addicted tumour cell will die while normal 'non-addicted' cells will be unaffected. A few of the major pathways are briefly discussed.

1.5 **Epidermal growth factor receptor signaling**

The EGFR (ErbB) family of tyrosine kinase receptors includes four members—EGFR, EGFR2 (HER2), EGFR3, and EGFR4. The receptors form homo- or heterodimers which results in receptor activation and subsequent activation of various signalling pathways including some involved in proliferation (RAS/MAPK), gene regulation (STAT signalling), invasion and metastasis, and evasion of apoptosis (PI3K/AKT). This pathway is activated in almost all solid tumours via a multitude of mechanisms, although SCLC appears to be an exception with almost all or all tumours lacking mutations or increased copy number changes in the key EGFR pathway genes. EGFR exhibits over-expression or aberrant activation in approximately 50–90% of NSCLCs with activating mutations occurring with or without amplification. Activating mutations, which are found with increased frequency in certain subsets of lung cancer patients, occur by three different types of somatic mutations in specific regions of the tyrosine kinase domain of the gene. Activating mutations are present in about 10% of Caucasians with lung cancer, and are more common in East Asians (30-40%). EGFR mutant tumours (primarily adenocarcinomas especially in those arising in never smokers of Asian ethnicity) are addicted to EGFR signalling. The mutant tumours initially are highly sensitive to EGFR tyrosine kinase inhibitors (TKIs). However, despite an initial response, patients treated with EGFR TKIs eventually develop resistance to TKIs which is linked (in approximately 50% tumours) to the acquisition of secondary mutations in the gene or to amplification of the MET oncogene.

1.6 The RAS/RAF/MEK/MAPK/MYC pathway

This pathway is one of the major arms of the EGFR signalling pathway. The best known method of activation is via activating mutations in the KRAS gene, which result in uncontrolled proliferation. These mutations occur in about 30% of adenocarcinomas arising in non-Asian ethnicities, especially smokers. Activating point mutations can confer oncogenic potential through a loss of intrinsic GTPase activity resulting in an inability to cleave GTP to GDP. BRAF mutations, less common than in melanomas or colorectal carcinomas, may also be present in a subset of adenocarcinomas. Of interest, EGFR, KRAS and BRAF mutations are almost entirely mutually exclusive, indicating that one of these mutations is sufficient for activation of the EGFR pathway. It has been suggested that the pathway is activated in smokers via KRAS mutations and in never smokers via EGFR mutations. However, the dominant activating mutation in about 50% of adenocarcinomas remains to be discovered.

The PI3K/AKT pathway which lies downstream of several receptor tyrosine kinases (RTKs) (such as EGFR) is a key regulator of cell proliferation, cell growth, and cell survival and is commonly activated in lung cancer through changes in several of its components including PI3K, PTEN, AKT, or EGFR or KRAS. In lung tumorigenesis, activation of the PI3K/AKT pathway is thought to occur early and results in cell survival through inhibition of apoptosis. Activation can occur through the binding of the SH2-domains of p85, the regulatory subunit of PI3K, to phosphotyrosine residues of activated RTKs. Alternatively, activation can occur via binding of PI3K to activated RAS. Mutation and more commonly, amplification of PIK3CA, which encodes the catalytic subunit of phosphatidylinositol 3-kinase (PI3K), occurs most commonly in squamous cell carcinomas. AKT, a serine/threonine kinase that acts downstream from PI3K can also have mutations that lead to pathway activation. One of the primary effectors of AKT is mTOR, a serine/threonine kinase involved in regulating proliferation, cell cycle progression, mRNA translation, cytoskeletal organization, and survival. The tumour suppressor PTEN, which negatively regulates the PI3K/AKT pathway via phosphatase activity on phosphatidylinositol 3, 4, 5-trisphosphate (PIP3), a product of PI3K is commonly suppressed in lung cancer by inactivating mutations or loss of expression.

1.6.1 **SOX2 and NKX2-1 (TITF1)—lung cancer lineage dependent oncogenes**

Genome-wide screens for DNA copy number changes in primary NSCLCs has led to the identification of multiple examples of amplification at 14q13.3 and 3q26.33, and functional analyses identified *NKX2-1* (also termed *TITF1*) and *SOX2* as the respective targets of these amplifications in lung cancer. *NKX2-1* encodes a lineage-specific transcription factor essential for branching morphogenesis in lung development and the formation of type II pneumocytes—the cells lining lung alveoli. *SOX2* amplification was identified specifically in squamous cell carcinomas and is required for normal esophageal squamous development. Amplification of tissue-specific transcription factors in cancer has been observed in *AR* in prostate cancer, *MITF* in melanoma, and *ESR1* in breast cancer. These findings have led to the development of a 'lineage-dependency' concept in tumours where the survival and progression of a tumour is dependent upon continued signalling through specific lineage pathways (i.e. continued abnormal expression of pathways involved in normal physiological cell development) rather than continued signalling through the pathway of oncogenic transformation as seen with oncogene addiction.

1.6.2 **EML4-ALK fusion proteins**

Oncogenic fusion proteins created by recurrent chromosomal translocations are generally not common in solid tumours such as lung cancer; however, recent studies indicate this infrequency may be attributable to the difficulties in detection. The fusion of PTK echinoderm microtubule-associated protein like-4 (EML4)-anaplastic lymphoma kinase (ALK) was recently associated with lung cancer, and occurs in approximately 7% of cases. Fusing with EML4 induces a significant transforming potential in ALK. While wildtype ALK is thought to undergo transient homodimerization in response with specific ligand binding, EML4-ALK is constitutively oligomerized resulting in persistent mitogenic signalling and ultimately malignant transformation. Additionally, EML4-ALK generally appears to be mutually exclusive to EGFR or KRAS mutations in NSCLC and is more common in never or former smokers.

1.6.3 **Tumour suppressor genes (TSGs) and growth inhibitory pathways**

Loss of TSG function is an important step in the lung carcinogenesis process and usually both alleles need to be inactivated. Generally, loss of heterozygosity (LOH) inactivates one allele through chromosomal deletion or translocation, and point mutation, epigenetic or transcriptional silencing inactivates the second allele. In lung cancer, commonly inactivated TSGs include *TP53*, *RB1*, *CDKN2A*, *FHIT*, *RASSF1A* and *PTEN*.

1.6.4 **The p53 pathway**

TP53 (17p13) encodes a phosphoprotein which prevents accumulation of genetic damage in daughter cells. In response to cellular stress, p53 induces the expression of downstream genes such as cyclin-dependent kinase (CDK) inhibitors which regulate cell cycle checkpoint signals, causing the cell to undergo G1 arrest and allowing DNA repair or apoptosis. p53 inactivating mutations are the most common alterations in cancer, especially lung cancer, where 17p13 frequently demonstrates hemizygous deletion and mutational inactivation in the remaining allele. Regulation of p53 can occur through the oncogene MDM2, which reduces p53 levels through degradation, and the p14^{ARF} isoform of *CDKN2A*, which acts as a tumour suppressor by inhibiting MDM2. As such, the genes that encode MDM2 and p14^{ARF} are altered in lung cancer with amplification of *MDM2* seen in 6% of NSCLCs and loss of p14^{ARF} expression in approximately 40% and 65% of NSCLCs and SCLCs, respectively. Restoration of p53 expression *in vivo* has been achieved with p53 gene therapy of lung cancer patients in a subpopulation of tumour cells.

1.6.5 **The CDKN2A/RB pathway**

The CDKN2A-RB1 pathway controls G1 to S phase cell cycle progression. Hypophosphorylated retinoblastoma (RB) protein, encoded by *RB1*, halts the G1/S phase transition by binding to the transcription factor E2F1. This tumour suppressing effect can be inhibited by hyperphosphorylation of RB by CDK-CCND1 complexes (complexes between CDK4 or CDK6 and CCND1), and in turn, formation of CDK-CCND1 complexes can be inhibited by CDNK2A. Nearly all constituents of the CDKN2A/RB pathway have been shown to be altered in lung cancer through mutations (*CDK4* and *CDKN2A*), deletions (*RB1* and *CDKN2A*), amplifications (*CDK4* and *CCDN1*), methylation silencing (*CDKN2A* and *RB1*), and phosphorylation (RB).

1.6.6 **Chromosome 3p TSGs**

Loss of one copy of chromosome 3p is one of the most frequent and early events in human cancer, found in 96% of lung tumours and 78% of lung preneoplastic lesions. Mapping of this loss identified several genes with functional tumour suppressing capacity including *FHIT* (3p14.2), *RASSF1A*, *TUSC2* (also called *FUS1*), and semaphorin family members *SEMA3B* and *SEMA3F* (all at 3p21.3), and *RARβ* (3p24). In addition to LOH or allele loss, some of these 3p genes (*FHIT*, *RASSF1A*, *SEMA3B* and *RAR*) often exhibit decreased expression in lung cancer cells by means of epigenetic mechanisms such as promoter hypermethylation. Additionally, *FHIT*, *RASSF1A*, *TUSC2*, and *SEMA3B* will reduce growth when re-introduced into lung cancer cells. *FHIT*, located in the most common fragile site in the human genome (*FRA3B*), has been shown to induce apoptosis in lung cancer.

RASSF1A can induce apoptosis, as well as stabilize microtubules, and affect cell cycle regulation. The tumour suppressing effect of *TUSC2* is thought to occur through inhibition of protein tyrosine kinases such as EGFR, PDGFR, c-Abl, c-Kit, and AKT as well as inhibition of MDM2-mediated degradation of p53. The candidate TSG *SEMA3B* encodes a secreted protein which can decrease cell proliferation and induce apoptosis when re-expressed in lung, breast and ovarian cancer cells in part, by inhibiting the AKT pathway. Another family member, *SEMA3F* may inhibit vascularization and tumorigenesis by acting on VEGF and ERK1/2 activation and *RAR* exerts its tumour suppressing function by binding retinoic acid, thereby limiting cell growth and differentiation.

1.6.7 **LKB1**

The serine/threonine kinase LKB1 (also called STK11) is inactivated in ~30% of lung cancers and often correlates with KRAS activation, resulting in the promotion of cell growth. It functions as a TSG by regulating cell polarity, differentiation, and metastasis and can regulate cell metabolism. It has also been reported to inhibit the mTOR pathway.

1.6.8 **Epigenetic regulation**

Genetic abnormalities are associated with changes in the DNA sequence, however epigenetic events may lead to changes in gene expression without any changes in the DNA sequence and therefore, importantly, the latter are potentially reversible. Aberrant promoter hypermethylation is an epigenetic change that occurs early in lung tumorigenesis and is found both in genes that normally undergo methylation in response to ageing, as well as in genes that normally remain unmethylated regardless of age. Gains of DNA methylation in a normally unmethylated promoter region of a gene results in silencing of gene transcription and is therefore a common method for the inactivation of tumour suppressor genes. In lung cancer, many genes have been found to be silenced by promoter hypermethylation (summarized in Table 1.1). They include genes involved in tumour suppression, tissue invasion, DNA repair, detoxification of tobacco carcinogens, and differentiation. Recent advances in whole-genome microarray profiling have allowed researchers to globally study DNA methylation patterns in lung cancer, the results of which have led to suggestions that the role of methylation in lung tumorigenesis has been underestimated. Restoration of expression of epigenetically silenced genes is a new targeted therapeutic approach. Histone deacetylation is an example of epigenetic change that can inhibit gene expression. Histone deacetylase inhibitors (HDACs) are being studied for the treatment of lung cancer and function by reversing gene silencing by inhibiting histone deacetylation (Table 1.2).

Table 1.1 The hallmarks of lung cancer

Hallmark of lung cancer	Major genes or pathways
Self-sufficiency of growth signals (oncogene activation)	EGFR signalling (EGFR, HER2, BRAF, KRAS, MEK) PIK3 pathway (PIK3CA, PTEN)
Insensitivity to antigrowth signals (tumour suppressor inactivation)	TP53, RB1, CDH1 (e-cadherin), CDH13, CDKN2A (p16), DAPK1, GSTP1, LKB1 (STK11), RAR, RASSF1A, FHIT, MGMT, TCF21
Evasion of programmed cell death (apoptosis)	AKT1, mTOR, Survivin, BCL2
Limitless replicative potential	Activation of telomerase, hTERT
Sustained angiogenesis	VEGF, VEGFR,
Tissue invasion and metastasis	TIMP3, MMP9

The list is not intended to be exhaustive, but for each hallmark some of the well-known genes involved in lung cancer pathogenesis are listed. As many of the pathways and genes interact with multiple others, their listing in one category is arbitrary.

Hanahan and Weinberg described the 'hallmarks of cancer' as six essential alterations in cell physiology that collectively dictate malignant growth. The major genes or pathways involved in these pathways in the pathogenesis of lung cancer are indicated.

Table 1.2 Targets for personalized medicine

- EGFR
- ERBB2 (HER2)
- KRAS
- BRAF
- mTOR
- MEK
- VEGF
- KIT
- BCL2
- SRC
- The Proteosome
- The Epigenome
- Telomerase
- FUS1
- TP53

The above is a list of lung cancer targets for personalized medicine currently in clinical use or in trials. The list is not exhaustive and many more potential targets will probably be tested in the not too distant future. Note, over half of the targets are in the EGFR signalling pathway.

1.6.9 **MicroRNA-mediated regulation of lung cancer**

MicroRNAs (miRNAs) are a recently identified class of non-protein encoding small RNAs present in the genomes of plants and animals. Ranging in size from 20–25 nucleotides, miRNAs are small RNA molecules that are capable of regulating gene expression by either direct cleavage of a targeted mRNA or inhibiting translation by interacting with the 3' untranslated region (UTR) of a target mRNA. They are considered to play an important role in the pathogenesis of cancer—as either oncogenes or TSGs—due to abnormal expression found in several types of cancer, including lung cancer. Additionally, more than 50% of miRNAs are located in cancer-associated genomic regions or fragile sites.

As observed for analyses on mRNA, protein and methylation patterns in lung cancer, miRNA microarrays have enabled the identification of many lung cancer-associated miRNAs. One of the most widely-studied miRNAs in lung cancer is the *let-7* miRNA family. Functioning as a tumour suppressor, it has been shown to regulate N-RAS, K-RAS and HMGA2 via binding to the let-7 binding sites in their respective 3' UTRs. It is frequently under-expressed in lung tumours, particularly NSCLC, compared to normal lung, and decreased expression has also been associated with poor prognosis. Induction of *let-7* miRNA expression has been found to inhibit growth *in vitro* and reduce tumour development in a murine model of lung cancer. In addition to *let-7*, other miRNAs with suggested tumour suppressing effects in lung cancer include *miR-126*, *miR-29a/b/c*, *miR-1*, and recently, *miR-128b* was reported to be a direct regulator of EGFR with frequent LOH occurring in NSCLC cell lines. Oncogenic miRNAs found to be over-expressed in lung cancer include the *miR-17-92* cluster of seven miRNAs (with suggested targets that include PTEN and RB), *miR-205*, *miR-21*, and *miR-155*.

1.6.10 **Lung cancer stem cells and Hedgehog, Notch and Wnt Signalling**

Lung cancer appears to have a 'cancer stem cell' component and it is likely this is regulated by stem cell signalling pathways. The Hedgehog (HH), Wnt and Notch signalling pathways are important in normal lung development—specifically progenitor cell development and pulmonary organogenesis—however, they are now also being studied in regard to their role in tumour development. These signalling pathways are thought to be involved in the regulation of stem/progenitor cell self-renewal and maintenance, and while this process is normally a tightly regulated process, genes that comprise these pathways are often mutated in human cancers, leading to abnormal activation of downstream effectors. In relation to cancer treatment, cancer stem cells are of great importance because they are thought to be resistant to cytotoxic therapies. If correct, this presents a need for effective therapies against these self-renewal signalling pathways.

In the HH pathway, increased signalling results in activation of the GLI oncogenes (GLI1, GLI2, and GLI3) that can regulate gene transcription. The HH signalling pathway was originally shown to have persistent activation in SCLC with high expression of SHH, PTCH, and GLI1 but an important role in NSCLC was also recently demonstrated. The Notch signalling pathway is important in cell fate determination but can also promote and maintain survival in many human cancers. A recent study in mammary stem cells suggests the cytokine IL-6 may function as a regulator of self renewal in normal and tumour mammary stem cells through the Notch pathway through upregulation of the Notch-3 receptor, which is expressed in ~40% of resected lung cancers. The multifunctional cytokine IL-6 is involved in activation of JAK family of tyrosine kinases, which in turn activate multiple pathways through signalling molecules such as STAT3, MAPK, and PI3K. In lung adenocarcinomas, activated mutant EGFR has also been shown to induce levels of IL-6 leading to activation of STAT3. The Wnt pathway has critical roles in organogenesis, cancer initiation, and progression, and maintenance of stem cell pluripotency. In NSCLC, studies have found dysregulation of Wnt pathway members such as Wnt1, Wnt2 and Wnt7a, as well as upregulation of Wnt pathway agonists (Dvl proteins, LEF1, and Ruvb11) and underexpression or silencing of antagonists (WIF-1, sFRP1, CTNNBIP1, and WISP2)

1.6.11 **Human papilloma virus-mediated lung cancer**

Human papilloma virus (HPV) has been identified in tumours from many organs, not just gynecological tumours. Nearly thirty years ago it was suggested to be a risk factor for lung cancer, particularly squamous cell carcinoma and since then, many studies have investigated the role of HPV in lung cancer and have reported considerable geographical variation. A recent meta-analysis of 53 publications comprising 4,508 cases found the mean incidence of HPV in lung cancer was 25% and was detected in all subtypes of lung cancer, not just squamous cell. Studies from Europe and America had a lower incidence of 15–17% while Asian lung cancer cases reported a mean incidence of 38%. This observed high penetrance of HPV in lung cancer suggests more research is required to elucidate its role in lung cancer pathogenesis; however, considering the significant variation observed between studies of cases from the same geographical location subsequent studies will need to have a large sample and a detailed study design.

1.7 **Summary**

Over the past decade, research into the biology of lung cancer, led by the development of global approaches for the analysis of expression, copy-number, methylation, microRNAs, and SNPs have elucidated many of the basic genetic and epigenetic mechanisms underlying lung cancer development and progression. Functional characterization of genetic alterations and the signalling pathways with which they interact, has enabled the development of targeted therapies for the treatment of lung cancer. Improvements in the pathological diagnosis and classification of lung cancers, especially involving the use of small biopsies or cytological material, have resulted in further selection criteria for therapy selection. Through the integration of clinical and biological factors these findings have led to the first steps of ultimate goal of achieving personalized medicine for all or most patients with lung cancer.

Further reading

Engelman J.A. and Janne P.A. (2008) Mechanisms of acquired resistance to epidermal growth factor receptor tyrosine kinase inhibitors in non-small cell lung cancer. *Clin Cancer Res* **14**(10): 2895–9.

Saijo N. (2008) Advances in the treatment of non-small cell lung cancer. *Cancer Treat Rev* **34**(6): 521–6.

Sato M., Shames D.S., Gazdar A.F., Minna J.D. (2007) A translational view of the molecular pathogenesis of lung cancer. *J Thorac Oncol* **2**(4): 327–43.

Sharma S.V., Bell D.W., Settleman J., Haber D.A. (2007) Epidermal growth factor receptor mutations in lung cancer. *Nat Rev Cancer* **7**(3): 169–81.

Sun S., Schiller J.H., Gazdar A.F. (2007) Lung cancer in never smokers—a different disease. *Nat Rev Cancer* **7**(10): 778–90.

Chapter 2

Staging of lung cancer

Sofie De Craene, Kurt G. Tournoy,
and Jan P. van Meerbeeck

> **Key points**
> - The changes in the 7th edition of the UICC-TNM-classification will improve the alignment of stage with prognosis and in certain subsets also with treatment.
> - The 7th edition of the UICC-TNM-classification is recommended for the classification of NSCLC, SCLC and carcinoid tumours of the lung.
> - The new international Nodal Chart incorporates the concept of 'nodal zones' instead of stations. In the superior mediastinum, the midline moved from the anatomic midline to the left border of the trachea.
> - Systematic lobe specific nodal sampling is recommended in all cases in order to document complete resection, accurately define nodal staging and objectivate pN status. This implies sampling of at least 3 mediastinal stations including always the subcarinal one and 3 N1-nodes.
> - A standardized definition of visceral pleural invasion (VPI) has been incorporated into the 7th edition of TNM and includes the use of an elastic stain in the determination of VPI.

15

2.1 Staging classification of lung cancer

Lung cancer is among the commonest malignancies in the industrialized world and the leading cause of cancer deaths in both men and women. Unfortunately, lung cancer is often diagnosed at an advanced stage and its overall 5-year survival is only approximately 15% or less. However, patients diagnosed at an early stage experience a 5-year survival of up to 80%. Approximately half of all non-small-cell lung cancers (NSCLC) are either localized or locally advanced at the time of diagnosis. By contrast, small-cell lung cancers (SCLC) are metastatic in up to 75% of cases at diagnosis. Accurate clinical staging is critical for an appropriate selection of patients for surgery and/or multimodality therapy. Pathological staging guides the decision on adjuvant therapy, if any.

The staging of NSCLC is based upon the tumour node metastasis (TNM) staging system, which describes the primary tumour characteristics (T) and the presence or absence of regional lymph node involvement (N) and of distant metastasis (M). The combination of T, N, and M descriptors determines the overall disease stage (stage I to IV).

The Staging Committee of the International Association for the Study of Lung Cancer (IASLC) collected a large database and recommended changes for the seventh edition of the TNM-classification of malignant tumours. These recommendations are based on an extensive and validated analysis of the largest database to date. The proposed changes will improve the alignment of stage with prognosis and, in certain subsets, with treatment.

2.2 Summary of changes in the staging system (shaded in Table 2.1)

- The new staging system is recommended for the classification of NSCLC, SCLC and carcinoid tumours of the lung
- The T descriptors have been redefined:
  - T1 has been subclassified into T1a (< 2 cm in maximal diameter) and T1b (> 2 to 3 cm)
  - T2 has been subclassified into T2a (>3 to < 5 cm in size) and T2b (> 5 to 7 cm in size)
  - T2 (> 7 cm in size) has been reclassified as T3
  - Multiple tumour nodules in the same lobe have been reclassified from T4 to T3
  - Multiple tumour nodules in the same lung but a different lobe have been reclassified from M1 to T4
- The M classification has been redefined: M1 has been subdivided into M1a and M1b
  - Malignant pleural and pericardial effusions have been reclassified from T4 to M1a
  - Separate tumour nodules in the contralateral lung are considered M1a
  - M1b designates distant metastases in extrathoracic organs and non-regional lymph nodes

2.2.1 Definitions for T, N, and M descriptors according to the 7th edition

Table 2.1 Definitions for T, N and M descriptors (IASLC, 2009)	
T (Primary Tumour)	
TX	Primary tumour cannot be assessed, or tumour proven by the presence of malignant cells in sputum or bronchial washings but not visualized by imaging or bronchoscopy
T0	No evidence of primary tumour
Tis	Carcinoma in situ
T1	Tumour 3 cm in greatest dimension, surrounded by lung or visceral pleura, without bronchoscopic evidence of invasion more proximal than the lobar bronchus (i.e., not in the main bronchus)[a]
T1a	Tumour ≤2 cm in greatest dimension
T1b	Tumour > 2 cm but ≤3 cm in greatest diameter
T2	Tumour > 3 cm but ≤7 cm or tumour with any of the following features Involves main bronchus, ≥2 cm distal to the carina Invades visceral pleura beyond the elastic layer Associated with atelectasis or obstructive pneumonitis that extends to the hilar region but does not involve the entire lung
T2a	Tumour > 3 cm but ≤5 cm in greatest diameter[c]
T2b	Tumour > 5 cm but ≤7 cm in greatest diameter
T3	Tumour > 7 cm in greatest diameter or one that directly invades any of the following: chest wall (including superior sulcus tumours), diaphragm, phrenic nerve, mediastinal pleura, parietal pericardium; or tumour in the main bronchus < 2 cm distal to the carina[a] but without involvement of the carina; or associated atelectasis or obstructive pneumonitis of the entire lung or separate tumour nodule(s) in the same lobe
T4	Tumour of any size that invades any of the following: mediastinum, heart, great vessels[d], trachea, recurrent laryngeal nerve, esophagus, vertebral body, carina, separate tumour nodule(s) in a different ipsilateral lobe
N (Regional Lymph Nodes)	
NX	Regional lymph nodes cannot be assessed
N0	No regional lymph node metastases
N1	Metastasis in ipsilateral 'double digit' lymph nodes nodes, including involvement by direct extension
N2	Metastasis in ipsilateral 'single digit' lymph node(s)
N3	Metastasis in contralateral 'single or double digit' lymph nodes, or in the ipsilateral or contralateral scalene lymph node station, or any lymph node station 1

Table 2.1 *(Continued)*	
M (Distant Metastasis)	
MX	Distant metastasis cannot be assessed
M0	No distant metastasis
M1	Distant metastasis
M1a	Separate tumour nodule(s) in a contralateral lobe; tumour with pleural nodules or malignant pleural (or pericardial) effusion[b]
M1b	Distant metastasis

[a] The uncommon superficial spreading tumour of any size with its invasive component limited to the bronchial wall, which may extend proximally to the main bronchus, is also classified as T1a.

[b] Most pleural (and pericardial) effusions with lung cancer are due to tumour. In a few patients, however, multiple cytopathologic examinations of pleural (pericardial) fluid are negative for tumour, and the fluid is nonbloody and is not an exudate. Where these elements and clinical judgement dictate that the effusion is not related to the tumour, the effusion should be excluded as a staging element and the patient should be classified as T1, T2, T3 or T4.

[c] A tumour that crosses the fissure is considered at least T2a in the absence of features

[d] The great vessels include: aorta, superior vena cava, inferior vena cava, main pulmonary artery, intrapericardial segments of the trunk of the right and left pulmonary artery, intrapericardial segments of the superior and inferior right and left pulmonary veins.

2.2.2 The mediastinal lymph node map (IASLC, 2009)

The regional lymph nodes involved in lung cancer are described as follows (Figure 2.1A):

- N1 nodes: all lymph nodes found within the reflection of the visceral pleura, consisting of the so-called 'double digit' lymph node stations 10 (hilar), 11 (lobar), 12 (interlobar), 13 (segmental) and 14 (subsegmental)

- mediastinal nodes consist of the so-called 'single digit' lymph node stations 1 (supraclavicular, sternal noth and low cervical), 2 (upper paratracheal), 3 (prevascular or retrotracheal), 4 (lower paratracheal), 5 (aortic), 6 (subaortic), 7 (subcarinal), 8 (paraesophageal) and 9 (pulmonary ligament).

- the different lymph node stations are telescoped in zones (see Figure 2.1A), but the use of these zones is optional

- The anatomical and radiological landmarks of the different regional lymph node stations have been accurately defined (Figure 2.1B).

All other lymph node stations, e.g. cervical, axillary, inguinal, retroperitoneal, internal mammary, are considered non-regional and their invasion is classified as M1b. Low cervical lymph nodes are however, part of station 1 and their invasion hence classified as N3.

Figure 2.1A The IASLC lymph node map shown with the proposed amalgamation of lymph node levels into 'zones'. (IASLC, 2009, with permission)

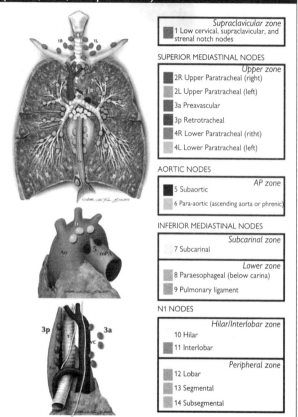

Supraclavicular zone
1 Low cervical, supraclavicular, and strenal notch nodes

SUPERIOR MEDIASTINAL NODES

Upper zone
2R Upper Paratracheal (right)

2L Upper Paratracheal (left)

3a Preavascular

3p Retrotracheal

4R Lower Paratracheal (ritht)

4L Lower Paratracheal (left)

AORTIC NODES

AP zone
5 Subaortic

6 Para-aortic (ascending aorta or phrenic)

INFERIOR MEDIASTINAL NODES

Subcarinal zone
7 Subcarinal

Lower zone
8 Paraesophageal (below carina)

9 Pulmonary ligament

N1 NODES

Hilar/Interlobar zone
10 Hilar

11 Interlobar

Peripheral zone
12 Lobar

13 Segmental

14 Subsegmental

Reproduced with permission from Peter Goldstraw, John Crowley, Kari Chansky, *et al.* (2007) The IASLC Lung Cancer Staging Project: Proposals for the Revision of the TNM Stage Groupings in the Forthcoming (Seventh) Edition of the TNM Classification of Malignant Tumours. *Journal of Thoracic Oncology*, 2(8):706–14.

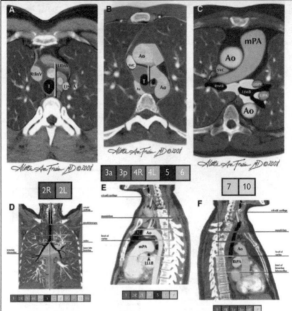

Figure 2.1B **Selected lymph node stations on representative CT scan sections**

Reproduced with permission from Valerie Rusch, Hisao Asamura, Hirokazu Watanabe, et al. (2009) The IASLC Lung Cancer Staging Project: A Proposal for a New International Lymph Node Map in the Forthcoming Seventh Edition of the TNM Classification for Lung Cancer. *Journal of Thoracic Oncology*, **4**(5): 568–577.

Table 2.2 **Stage grouping with corresponding median and 5-year overall survival by clinical and pathological stage, using the seventh edition of TNM (IASLC, 2009)**

	By clinical stage		By pathologic stage	
	Median	5-Year	Median	5-Year
IA	60 m	50%	119 m	73%
IB	43 m	43%	81 m	58%
IIA	34 m	36%	49 m	46%
IIB	18 m	25%	31 m	36%
IIIA	14 m	19%	22 m	24%
IIIB	10 m	7%	13 m	9%
IV	6m	2%	17%	13%

2.2.3 **Stage Grouping**

2.2.3.1 *Stage grouping of NSCLC according to UICC 7 (Figure 2.2)*

Figure 2.2 Stage grouping of NSCLC according to UICC 7 (IASLC, 2009)

	M0	N0	N1	N2	N3
T1a		I A	II A	III A	III B
T1b		I A	II A	III A	III B
T2a		I B	II A	III A	III B
T2b		II B	II B	III A	III B
T3		II A	III A	III A	III B
T4		III A	III A	III A	III B
M1a, b	IV	IV	IV	IV	IV

2.2.3.2 *SCLC*

The two stage system originally introduced by the Veterans' Affairs Lung Study Group (VALSG) has been widely used because of its simplicity and clinical utility:

• Limited stage was defined as any extension confined to the ipsilateral hemithorax and within a single radiotherapy port (corresponding to TNM stages I to IIIB).

• Extensive stage was defined as any extension beyond 'limited', corresponding to TNM stages IV and some IIIB)

This distinction is clinically relevant, since patients with limited disease are generally treated with combined modality therapy, while those with extensive stage disease receive chemotherapy alone. A so-called 'very limited' substage includes patients with T1-2N0 who can proceed to resection. As mentioned, the use of the seventh UICC-TNM classification is presently recommended in SCLC.

2.2.4 **Clinical and pathological staging**

- Clinical staging (cTNM): based on evidence acquired before treatment, including physical examination, imaging studies and staging procedures.

- Pathological staging (pTNM): uses the evidence acquired before treatment, supplemented or modified by the additional evidence acquired during and after surgery, particularly from pathological examination. It is not a prerequisite that the primary tumour has been removed completely to obtain a pT. However in those cases, a biopsy must have confirmed the highest T-status. Similarly, pN can be used whenever there is biopsy confirmation of nodal disease at any level (pN1-3) or there is confirmation of the highest N-category (pN3).

- The extent of regional lymph node involvement in patients with lung cancer is an important prognostic factor and influences therapeutic strategies. Systematic lobe specific nodal sampling or dissection is recommended (Table 2.3) in all cases by the UICC in order to document pN0. This implies removal or sampling of at least 3 mediastinal nodes (including the subcarinal station) and 3 hilar and/or interlobar nodes. Omission of lobe specific mediastinal lymph node sampling is only acceptable for peripheral squamous T1 tumours, if hilar and interlobar nodes are negative on frozen section examination.

Selected lymph node sampling is justified to prove nodal involvement whenever a resection is not possible.

- If gross inspection of the lymph node does not detect any macroscopic invasion, 2 mm slices of the nodes in the longitudinal plane are recommended. Routine search for micrometastases or isolated tumour cells (ITC) in hematoxylin-eosin negative nodes is currently not advised. Cases with ITC in the LN should be classified as pN0. In addition, the connotations N0 (i+) or N0 (mol+) may now be used to indicate that these ITC were detected by immunohistochemistry or molecular techniques, respectively.

- A standardized definition and subclassification of visceral pleural invasion (VPI) has been incorporated into the 7th edition of TNM with recommendations on the use of elastic stains in the

Table 2.3 Lobe specific intraoperative lymph node sampling	
Lobe resected	**Mediastinal lymph nodes systematically sampled**
Right upper and middle lobe	2R, 4R, and 7
Right lower lobe	4R, 7, 8, and 9
Left upper lobe	5, 6, and 7
Left lower lobe	7, 8, and 9

determination of VPI (Figure 2.3). VPI is defined as any invasion beyond the elastic layer. PL0 represents either tumour within the subpleural lung parenchyma or invading superficially into the pleural connective tissue beneath the elastic layer. If a tumour invades beyond the elastic layer it is classified PL1. Tumours that invade to the pleural surface are PL2 and those that invade into any component of the parietal pleura are PL3. PL0 is not regarded as a T descriptor and the T category should be assigned on other features. PL1 and PL2 indicate VPI and are coders for a T2 descriptor. PL3 indicates invasion of the parietal pleura and is a T3 descriptor. If the PL category is unknown, PLx can be used.

- R-denominator: a resection is considered complete (R0), whenever both following microscopic criteria are met: absence of tumour in all resection margins and in the highest systematically resected mediastinal lymph node station. Whenever one of those criteria is not met, a R1-resection is present. If macroscopic tumour is left in place, the resection is considered R2. When the R-denominator is not assessable or no systematic lymph node sampling is performed, Rx can be used.

Figure 2.3 Descriptor of pleural invasion PL (see text)

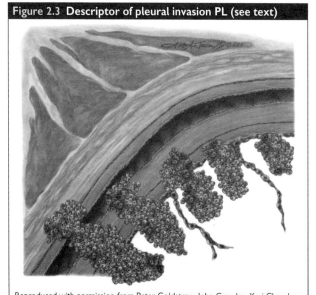

Reproduced with permission from Peter Goldstraw, John Crowley, Kari Chansky, et al. (2007) The IASLC Lung Cancer Staging Project: Proposals for the Revision of the TNM Stage Groupings in the Forthcoming (Seventh) Edition of the TNM Classification of Malignant Tumours, *Journal of Thoracic Oncology*, **2**(8):706–14.

2.2.5 **Special situations**

- Multiple synchronous tumours should be considered separate primary lung cancers, and each should be staged separately. These include multiple synchronous tumours of different histological types or two tumours of the same histological type in separate lobes with no evidence of either extrathoracic disease, or of mediastinal nodal metastases or of nodal metastases within a common nodal drainage (e.g. involved interlobar nodes with right upper and lower lobe tumours of the same histology).

- Vocal cord paralysis resulting from the involvement of the recurrent branch of the vagus nerve may be related to direct extension of the primary tumour. In that case, a classification of T4 is recommended. If the primary tumour is peripheral, vocal cord paralysis is usually related to the presence of N2 disease and should be classified as such.

- Pancoast tumours relates to the symptom complex caused by a tumour arising in the superior sulcus of the lung involving the inferior branches of the brachial plexus (C8 and/or T1) and, in some cases, the stellate ganglion (with Horner syndrome). Some superior sulcus tumours are more anteriorly located, and cause fewer neurological symptoms but encase subclavian vessels. If there is evidence of invasion of the vertebral body or spinal canal, encasement of the subclavian vessels, or unequivocal involvement of the superior branches of the brachial plexus (C8 or above), the tumour is classified as T4. If no criteria for T4 disease pertain, the tumour is classified as T3.

- Paraneoplastic syndromes or elevated serum tumour markers (CEA, NSE) are not associated with tumour extent and their presence does not obviate the need for complete staging.

2.3 **Staging procedures**

The recommendations by the American College of Chest Physicians (ACCP) represents the most comprehensive evidence-based summary currently available (Silvestri, 2007; Detterbeck, 2007). A staging algorithm based on this evidence is proposed for NSCLC (Figure 2.4).

Patients with lung cancer should be staged with great care and accuracy because the treatment options and prognosis differ significantly by stage. Once there is no evidence for haematogenous metastasis, the mediastinum should be investigated.

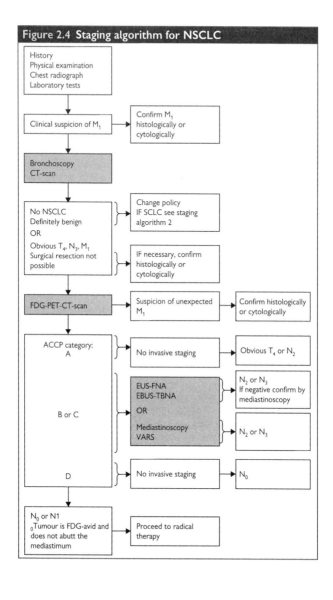

Figure 2.4 Staging algorithm for NSCLC

2.3.1 **For disseminated disease**

The most common metastatic sites are the brain, bones, adrenal glands, contralateral lung, liver, pericardium, kidneys, and subcutaneous tissues. However, virtually any organ can be a site of metastatic disease.

In the case of a patient with NSCLC, without clinical suspicion of distant metastasis, one will perform an FDG- PET-scan in order to detect occult distant metastasis in 10–15% of patients. Solitary extrathoracic sites of FDG-PET avidity should be confirmed, preferably by biopsy if corresponding to an anatomic substrate. FDG-PET scan is insufficiently sensitive to detect metastatic foci smaller than 4 mm. The role of FDG-PET scan in the evaluation of distant metastases appears to be the greatest for adrenal and bone metastases. FDG-PET-scan is not useful for the detection of brain metastases due to the high glucose uptake of normal brain tissue. As 10–15% of patients with clinical stage III have occult brain metastasis, a contrast enhanced CT or MRI of the brain is hence recommended.

The FDG-PET scan is potentially useful in the staging of SCLC. However, there is less information on FDG-PET scan in the staging of SCLC and controversy remains about its superior efficacy to discriminate between extensive and limited stages. For SCLC (Figure 2.5), a cost-effective algorithm has been developed by Richardson *et al.* (1993). The few cases that proceed to resection are best staged according to the NSCLC guidelines.

2.3.2 **Intrathoracic/mediastinal staging**

2.3.2.1 *Non-invasive staging of the mediastinum*

- A spiral CT scan with contrast enhancement allows accurate measuring of the T size, demonstration of atelectasis, is specific for T3 and T4 invasion; but non-specific for the differentiation between benign and malignant lymph nodes. Separate tumour nodule(s) in a contralateral lobe; tumour with pleural nodules or pleural (or pericardial) effusion (M1a) are also readily demonstrated.

- A FDG-PET scan is more accurate than CT for detecting malignant lymph node disease and for detecting pleural involvement and malignant pleural effusion. It has a high sensitivity and a reasonable specificity for differentiating benign from malignant lesions as small as 1 cm. Limited data exist for lesions less than 1 cm in diameter. False positives can occur with infection and inflammation. Therefore, any positive finding on a FDG-PET scan of the mediastinum should be histologically or cytologically confirmed to avoid denying patients potentially curative surgery. False negative results can occur whenever atelectasis due to the primary tumour obscures the mediastinal lymph nodes.

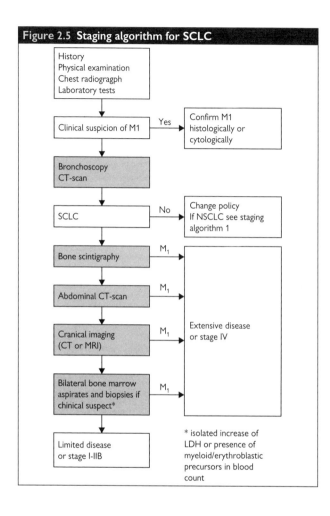

Figure 2.5 Staging algorithm for SCLC

History
Physical examination
Chest radiogragph
Laboratory tests

↓

Clinical suspicion of M1 —Yes→ Confirm M1 histologically or cytologically

↓

Bronchoscopy
CT-scan

↓

SCLC —No→ Change policy If NSCLC see staging algorithm 1

↓ M₁

Bone scintigraphy →

↓ M₁

Abdominal CT-scan →

↓ M₁

Cranical imaging (CT or MRI) →   Extensive disease or stage IV

↓ M₁

Bilateral bone marrow aspirates and biopsies if chinical suspect* →

↓

Limited disease or stage I-IIB

* isolated increase of LDH or presence of myeloid/erythroblastic precursors in blood count

- Integrated FDG-PET/CT provides simultaneous metabolic and anatomical information. It is generally agreed that FDG-PET/CT improves the accuracy of the T-descriptor and is to be preferred for intrathoracic staging.
- There is no place for routine thoracic MRI in lung cancer staging although there might be a benefit for selected patients with a superior sulcus tumour for the exact delineation and extent of malignant invasion in the spine and nervous structures.

2.3.2.2 *Invasive staging of the mediastinal lymph nodes*

For central tumours, a bronchoscopy is necessary to assess the proximal extent of the tumour besides allowing a diagnostic biopsy.

The gold standard of mediastinal staging is considered mediastinoscopy, either by a transcervical or a parasternal approach. Thoracotomy, either exploratory or video assisted (VATS), is sometimes necessary for accurate mediastinal staging in special circumstances.

In recent years, minimally invasive staging with endoscopic ultrasound techniques was shown to be an accurate alternative for invasive mediastinal surgical staging and can be obtained by either transoesophageal endoscopic ultrasound with fine needle-aspiration (EUS-FNA), endobronchial ultrasound with transbronchial needle aspiration (EBUS-TBNA) or a combination of both.

The ACCP guidelines propose the following work-up, according to 4 radiological presentations with different a priori suspicion of mediastinal involvement (Figure 2.6).

- Patients in category A are defined as patients in whom the tumour mass directly invades the mediastinum such that discrete lymph nodes cannot be distinguished or measured. In these patients, radiographic assessment of the mediastinal stage is sufficient, and no invasive confirmation is warranted ('obvious T4'). This holds also for patients in whom vocal cord paralysis is found during bronchoscopy, suggesting a direct invasion of the recurrent nerve. In case of doubt, a selected patient can be proposed an exploratory thoracotomy to verify the resectability.

- Patients in category B have one or more enlarged (short axis ≥10 mm) mediastinal lymph nodes. In this group, invasive confirmation is recommended and many techniques (EUS-FNA, EBUS-TBNA, mediastinoscopy) are equally reasonable. Negative fine needle aspirates should however always be confirmed because the negative predictive value of these techniques does not warrant immediate thoracotomy. This recommendation is unrelated to the FDG-PET findings as it takes into account a 20–28% false negative rate of PET-CT in those patients.

- Patients in category C have either a central lung tumour (within the proximal one third of the hemithorax) or clinical N1 tumour (enlarged or with FDG uptake) but a normal mediastinum (no enlarged lymph nodes, no FDG uptake). In these patients, invasive staging of the mediastinum is needed and in general a mediastinoscopy is suggested although EUS-FNA and/or EBUS-TBNA may be reasonable alternatives if non-diagnostic results are followed by mediastinoscopy. The latter relates to the negative predictive value of the minimally invasive fine needle techniques,

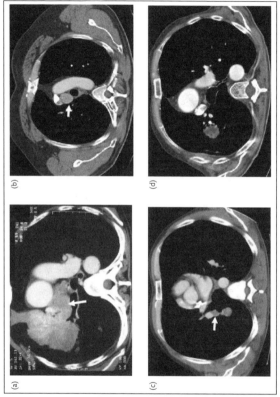

Figure 2.6 Categories of mediastinal lymph node involvement in NSCLC patients (see text) (Detterbeck, 2007)

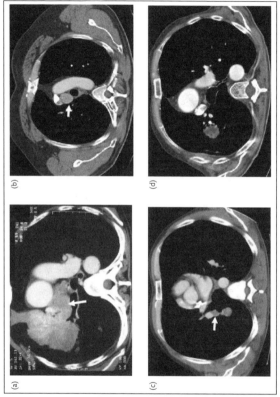

but it is presently not clear if the negative predictive value of mediastinoscopy after a negative EUS-FNA or EBUS-TBNA really contributes to a better clinical staging in these particular patients. On the other hand, ruling out malignant mediastinal invasion is important in these patients, and a thorough preoperative mediastinal lymph node sampling is the only valid way to achieve this. Both fine needle techniques are as single procedures not suited to do a systematic sampling, and by consequence, it seems logical to propose a mediastinoscopy in these situations. Whether combined procedures (EUS-FNA + EBUS-TBNA) are an alternative is currently under investigation.

• The patients in category D have a peripheral lung lesion (outer two thirds of the hemithorax) and both a normal mediastinum and hilar lymph nodes (<1cm). The false negative rates for mediastinal invasion are 9% for T1 tumours, and are as low as 5% in case FDG-PET shows no FDG-avidity in the mediastinal nodes. By consequence, invasive staging of the mediastinum is not recommended for these patients.

Further reading

Detterbeck F.C., Jantz M.A., Wallace M., Vansteenkiste J., Silverstri G.A.: American College of Psychiatrists (2007). Invasive mediastinal staging of lung cancer: ACCP evidence-based clinical practice guidelines (2nd Edition). *Chest* **132** (Suppl): S220.

Goldstraw P., Crowley J., Chansky K., *et al.* (2007). The IASLC lung cancer staging project: proposals for the revision of the TNM stage groupings in the forthcoming (seventh) edition of the TNM classification of malignant tumours. *J Thorac Oncol* **2**(8): 706–14.

International Association for the Study of Lung Cancer (IASLC) (2009). *Staging Manual in Thoracic Oncology*, Ed. P. Goldstraw. Editorial Rx Press, Orange Park, FL, USA.

Lardinois D., De Leyn P., Van Schil P. (2006). ESTS guidelines for intraoperative lymph node staging in non-small cell lung cancer. *Eur J Cardiothorac Surg* **30**: 787–92.

Richardson G.E., Venzon D.J., Edison M. (1993). Application of an algorithm for staging small-cell lung cancer can save one third of the initial evaluation costs. *Arch Intern Med* **153**: 328–37.

Sivestri G.A., Gould M.K., Margolis M.K. (2007). Noninvasive staging of non-small cell lung cancer: ACCP evidenced-based clinical practice guidelines (2nd Edition). *Chest* **123** (Suppl): S178–201.

Chapter 3

Systemic therapy for early-stage NSCLC

Benjamin Besse and Jean-Charles Soria

> ## Key points
> - Data supporting the use of adjuvant chemotherapy are more conclusive and robust than those for induction chemotherapy, although efficacy may be comparable
> - Patients under 75 years, PS 0 or 1 without surgical complications were included in the peri-operative prospective trials
> - Cisplatin-based chemotherapy is standard in radically-resected stage II and IIIA patients
> - Cisplatin-based chemotherapy is optional for stage IB patients (in particular those superior to 4 cm) and is not recommended for stage IA patients
> - Adjuvant chemotherapy should begin within 2 months after surgery and 3 to 4 cycles are recommended (cumulative dose of cisplatin from 240 to 400 mg/m²)
> - Vinorelbine-cisplatin is the most validated regimen in randomized trials while carboplatin should only be favoured in case of contraindications to cisplatin.

Aggressive surgical management of non–small-cell lung cancer (NSCLC) patients results in a 5-year survival rate ranging from 73% for pathologic stage IA to 25% for stage IIIA. The survival rates for a given clinical stage are much lower than those for the corresponding surgical/pathologic stage due to the preoperative staging that often underestimates the extent of the disease (particularly if positron-emission tomography and mediastinoscopy are not used) Given these poor survival rates associated with treatment by surgery alone, the use of induction or adjuvant systemic treatment have been investigated for years. In the last individual data based (IPD) meta-analysis from IGR-MRC on adjuvant treatment, reported in 2007, a 4% absolute improvement of the 5-year survival rate (HR = 0.87; 95% CI, 0.81 to 0.93; P = 0.0000001) resulted from the analysis of data of 8,147 patients. Cisplatin-based regimen emerged as the best adjuvant chemotherapeutic option. Adjuvant chemotherapy is better validated than induction chemotherapy, although their efficacy may be comparable. The most recent meta-analysis regarding induction chemo-therapy on 1,507 patients reported a hazard ratio of 0.88 (95% CI = 0.76–1.01; P = .07).

3.1 Adjuvant trials

Most of the early adjuvant trials were small and underpowered to detect a survival benefit. In the late 1990s, larger adjuvant trials were performed, three of which demonstrated a statistically significant survival benefit from cisplatin-based chemotherapy in stage I-III NSCLC (Table 3.1). Absolute 5-year survival differences ranged from 4% to 15% (HR = 0.69 to 0.86). On the basis of these results, postoperative cisplatin-based chemotherapy is now widely accepted as the standard treatment for patients with NSCLC. This option may be offered to those who fit the inclusion criteria of these positive trials: age under 75, performance status (PS) of 0 or 1, absence of surgical complications. The Lung Adjuvant Cisplatin Evaluation (LACE) meta-analysis pooled individual data from 4,584 patients included in five recent randomized adjuvant cisplatin-based chemotherapy trials. With a median follow-up of 5.1 years (range 3.1 to 5.9 years), the 5-year absolute benefit with chemotherapy was 5.3% (HR = 0.89; 95% CI, 0.82 to 0.96; P=0.005). Of interest, the benefit is also present for patients over 70.

Uracil plus tegafur (UFT) was evaluated as an adjuvant treatment in Japanese populations. The data for 2,003 patients from six studies were pooled in a meta-analysis based on individual data. Most of the patients had an adenocarcinoma (83.8%), a stage I NSCLC (98.8% had pathological T1 or T2 and 96% had no nodal involvement) and received adjuvant UFT for 1 year (35%) or 2 years (65%). The 5- and 7-year OS rates in the surgery plus UFT group were 81.8% and 76.5% vs 77.2% and 69.5% in the surgery-alone group (HR 0.74, 95% CI 0.61–0.88, P=0.001). The feasibility and benefit of adjuvant UFT in non-Asian populations is unknown. Its use cannot currently be recommended in caucasian populations.

3.2 Neoadjuvant trials

No IPD meta-analyses of neoadjuvant therapy trials have previously been carried out, and available studies based on abstracted or pooled data are less useful. Burdett *et al.* included in their meta-analysis 7 of the 12 eligible randomized trials (5 trials were excluded,

Table 3.1 Recent randomized platin-based adjuvant trials and meta-analyses

Trial	No. of patients	Stage	Chemotherapy	5-year benefit (%)	Hazard Ratio [95 % CI]	P
ALPI (Scagliotti et al. 2003)	1,209	I-IIIA	MVdP*	3	0.96 [0.81 to 1.13]	0.589
IALT (Arriagada et al. 2009)	1,867	I-IIIA	VincaP or EP*	4	0.91 [0.81 to 1.02]† 0.86 [0.76 to 0.98]	0.1† 0.03
BLT (Waller et al. 2004)	381	I-IIIA	Platin-based*	-2 (2 yrs)	1.02 [0.77 to 1.35]	0.90
BR10 (Butts et al. 2010)	482	IB-II	VnrP	11 15	0.78 [0.61 to 0.99] 0.69 [0.52 to 0.91]	0.04† 0.014
CALGB (Strauss et al. 2008)	344	IB	PacCb	2	0.83 [0.64 to 1.08] 0.62 [0.44 to 0.89]	0.125† 0.014
ANITA (Douillard et al. 2006)	840	IB-IIIA	VnrP*	9	0.8 [0.66 to 0.96]	0.017
NATCH (Massuti et al. 2009)	420	IA(T>2cm), IB, II and T3N1	PacCb	1.5	0.99 [0.75 to 1.3]	0.93
LACE (Pignon et al. 2008)	4,584	I-IIIA	Cisplatin-based*	5	0.89 [0.82 to 0.96]	0.005

Abbreviations: EP, etoposide/cisplatin; ALPI, Adjuvant Lung Project Italy; MVdP, mitomycin/vindesine/cisplatin; IALT, International Adjuvant Lung Trial; VincaP, vinorelbine, vindesine, or vinblastine/cisplatin; BLT, Big Lung Trial; BR10: from NCIC-CTG, National Institute of Canada Clinical Trials Group; VnrP, vinorelbine/cisplatin; CALGB, Cancer and Leukemia Group B; PacCb, paclitaxel/carboplatin; ANITA, Adjuvant Navelbine International Trialist Association; LACE, Lung Adjuvant Ciplatin Evaluation; * optional adjuvant radiotherapy; †updated data as the data that could be extracted from the published studies were insufficient) (Table 3.2). Two trials used carboplatin-based chemotherapy, while all others were cisplatin-based chemotherapy combinations. A total of 988 patients were included. The authors found that preoperative chemotherapy improved survival, with a hazard ratio of 0.82 (95% CI = 0.69–0.97, P = .02). This is equivalent to an absolute benefit of 6% at 5 years. This meta-analysis was recently updated. With a total of 1,507 patients, a hazard ratio of 0.88 (95% CI = 0.76–1.01, P = .07) was obtained, equivalent to an absolute improvement in survival of 5% at 5 years, nevertheless it did not reach statistical significance.

3.3 Chemotherapy regimens

3.3.1 Cisplatin vs carboplatin

In the metastatic setting, the CISCA (cisplatin vs carboplatin) meta-analysis based on individual data for 2,968 patients concluded that the response rate to chemotherapy including cisplatin (30%) is higher than that to chemotherapy including carboplatin (24%), with an OR of 1.37 (P = 0.001). Carboplatin treatment was associated with a non-statistically significant increase in the hazard of mortality relative to treatment with cisplatin in the whole population (HR 1.07, 95% CI 0.99–1.15, P = 0.100), but this excess of risk became significant in the patients with nonsquamous tumours and those treated with third-generation chemotherapy. In the adjuvant setting, the only published adjuvant trial using carboplatin is the CALGB study (paclitaxel plus carboplatin). Its findings were negative but the study may be underpowered. The Intergroupe Francophone de Cancérologie Thoracique (IFCT) 0002 study randomized four cycles of preoperative chemotherapy versus two cycles of preoperative chemotherapy and two postoperative cycles, using either gemcitabine/cisplatin (GC) or paclitaxel/carboplatin (PC). In the 528 patients included, the response rates were similar after 2 cycles of both regimens (52% for GC, 49% for PC) and the 3-year survival did not differ (69.5% for GC, 67.9% for PC). Nevertheless, cisplatin should be the platinum compound of choice in the peri-operative setting unless there are medical contraindications to its use.

The activity of the agent combined with platinum was evaluated in the LACE analysis. The effect of adjuvant chemotherapy did not differ significantly (test for interaction, P = .10) for the drugs used even if the vinorelbine-cisplatin combination (HR = 0.80; 95% CI = 0.70–0.91) appeared somewhat superior to etoposide/vinca-alkaloid-cisplatin (0.93; 0.80–1.07), and other combinations (0.98; 0.84–1.14).

Trial	No. of Patients	Stage	Chemotherapy	ORR	Complete resection Rate (%) S/S+C	Hazard Ratio [95% CI]	P
Rosell et al., 1999	60	IIIA	MIP	60%	90/77	–	0.005
Roth et al., 1998	60	IIIA	CEP	35%	31/39	–	0.056
Depierre et al., 2002	373	IB-IIIA	MIP	64%	26/37	0.78 [0.60 to 1.02]	0.15
LU22 (Gillian et al., 2007)	519	I-IIIA	VnrP, GemP, MVdP, Doc/carbo	49%	80/82	1.02 [0.80 to 1.31]	0.86
Ch.E.S.T. (Scagliotti et al., 2008)	344	IB-IIIA	GemP	35%	–	0.63 [0.42 to 0.93]	0.005
NATCH (Massuti et al., 2009)	409	IA (T>2cm), IB, II and T3N1	PacCb	2.6	–	0.96 [0.84 to 1.1]	0.56
Berghmans et al., 2005	590	I-IIIA	Cisplatin-based	–	NR/NR	0.66 [0.48 to 0.93]	
Meta-analysis 2007 (Gilligan et al., 2007)	1,507	I-IIIA	Cisplatin-based	–	NR/NR	0.88 [0.76 to 1.01]	0.07

Table 3.2 Recent randomized platin-based induction trials and meta-analyses

Abbreviations: ORR, objective response rate; S, surgery; S+C induction chemotherapy and surgery; MIP, mitomycin/ifosfamide/cisplatin; CEP, etoposide/cisplatin/cyclophsphamide ; VnrP, vinorelbine/cisplatin; GemP, gemcitabine/cisplatin; MVdP, mitomycin/vindesine/cisplatin; Doc/carbo, docetaxel/carboplatin.

The number of cycles of chemotherapy range from 3 to 4 in the perioperative trials, but this is still a matter of debate. The IFCT 0002 trials showed that responses to neoadjuvant treatment did not differ after 2 or 4 cycles (50.6% and 50.9%, respectively).

3.4 **Benefit by stage**

In the adjuvant pooled-analysis LACE, patients were divided into approximately equal groups as a function of disease stage (IA: 8%, IB: 30%, II: 35%, III: 27%). The benefit was different for patients with different stages of disease (test for trend, P = .046). The hazard ratio was 1.41 (95% CI = 0.96–2.09) for stage IA, 0.93 (0.78–1.10) for stage IB, 0.83 (0.73–0.95) for stage II, and 0.83 (0.73–0.95) for stage III. These results therefore discourage the use of adjuvant chemotherapy in stage IA patients.

In the IGR-MRC individual patient meta-analysis, 65% of the patients had stage I disease, 16% had stage II, 17% had stage IIIA, and 1% had stage IIIB (with less than 1% unknown). Cisplatin-based chemotherapy (without UFT) was only used for 54% of the patients. Overall, adjuvant chemotherapy significantly increased the overall survival rate, with an absolute benefit at 5 years of 4% in all stages. Out of the 5,353 patients had a stage I disease (65% of the patients), including 2,010 stage IA patients. However, antimetabolite agents (in particular UFT) without cisplatin were used in eight trials, mainly in Asian populations and in stage I adenocarcinomas, reducing the relevance of this analysis. Adjuvant UFT may be an option in this highly selected population but adjuvant cisplatin-based chemotherapy is not routinely included in the management of stage IA disease.

The only large platin-based adjuvant trial focusing on patients with stage IB disease was the CALGB study which failed to show improvement in survival. Various explanations for the negative results of this study have been suggested, including paclitaxel plus carboplatin being less active than cisplatin-based doublets, and the low statistical power of the trial as a consequence of early discontinuation of recruitment. Subgroup analysis of the JBR.10, ANITA and CALGB trials suggested a benefit when the tumour was larger than 4 cm. As a consequence, the population eligible for the ongoing adjuvant chemotherapy trial ECOG 1505 includes stage I disease >4 cm.

3.5 **Compliance and toxicity**

The acute toxicity of platin-based chemotherapy is roughly similar in the perioperative and the metastatic settings, but the death rate ranges from 0 to 2% in the adjuvant trials (Table 3.3). The compliance is improved when chemotherapy is given preoperatively since adjuvant chemotherapy is dependent on the absence of surgical complications. Table 3.3 summarizes the compliance to chemotherapy in the main randomized phase III studies of induction and adjuvant chemotherapy. In the IFCT 0002 study, 90.4% of the patients received the four cycles in the arm 'four cycles of preoperative chemotherapy' compared to 75.2% in the arm 'two cycles of preoperative chemotherapy and two postoperative cycles'. Similar data come from the NATCH trial that compared 3 cycles of neoadjuvant or adjuvant paclitaxel/carboplatin to surgery alone. Of the 199 patients randomized in the induction arm, 90% received the 3 planned cycles against only 61% of the 210 patients in the adjuvant arm. Compliance to adjuvant chemotherapy might be improved by the use of less toxic agents, such as the cytotoxic drug pemetrexed (Alimta®) or targeted agents such as the EGFR inhibitor erlotinib (Tarceva®). This is currently being evaluated in prospective clinical trials such as the French IFCT0801 trial (TASTE).

3.6 Long-term toxicities

IALT, the largest cisplatin-based adjuvant study, was positive after a median follow up of 56 months but the significant effect was no longer present after a median follow up of 90 months (Table 3.1). The concerns regarding the long term benefit of chemotherapy were also raised by the final results of the adjuvant CALGB study that negatively confirmed the initially positive results (Table 3.1). One explanation of the fading effect of adjuvant NSCLC chemotherapy could be realated to toxicity of the cytotoxic agents. Late effects of cisplatin-containing chemotherapy regimens, particularly vascular disease, have been well characterized after treatment of testicular cancer. Regarding lung cancer patients, the high rate of comorbidity at baseline may induce more long-term chemotherapy-associated toxicity. A higher rate of non-cancer related deaths has been reported in IALT after five years of follow-up. However, the long term results of the JBR.10 trial and the ANITA trial (with a median follow up of more than 7 and 9 years respectively) show only a slight decrease of the adjuvant chemotherapy benefit, but this benefit remains significant.

3.7 Targeted therapies and biomarkers

The understanding of lung cancer biology may be exploited to help develop novel therapies. Approved drugs in the metastatic setting (EGFR inhibitors such as erlotinib and gefitinib and the antiangiogenic monoclonal antibody bevacizumab) are currently being tested in the

Table 3.3 Regimens, compliance and toxicity of described in recent randomized platin-based induction or adjuvant trials

	Trial	Regimen		No. of cycles	Compliance	RT	% death
		Platinum	Other				
Adjuvant	IALT (Arriagada et al., 2009)	Cis 80 to 120 mg/m² q3w or q4w	Vindesine 3 mg/m²/w* Vinblastine 4 mg/m²/w* Vinorelbine 30 mg/m²/w Etoposide 100 mg/m² d1, d2, d3	3 to 4	73% received . 240 mg/m² cisplatin	31%	0.8%
	ALPI (Scagliotti et al., 2003)	Cis 100 mg/m² q4w	Mitomycin C (8 mg/m² d1), Vindesine (3 mg/m² d1, d8)	3	69% received 3 cycles, 31% received full dose	70%	0.5%
	BR10 (Butts et al., 2009)	Cis 100 mg/m² q4w	Vinorelbine 25 mg/m²/w	4	58% received ≥3 cycles, 77% received a lower dose	0%	0.8%
	CALGB (Strauss et al., 2008)	Cb AUC6	Paclitaxel 200 mg/m²	4	86% received 4 cycles	0%	0%
	ANITA (Douillard et al., 2006)	Cis 100 mg/m² q4w	Vinorelbine 30 mg/m²/w	4	63% received >260 mg/m² cisplatin	28%	2%
	NATCH (Massuti et al., 2009)	Cb AUC6	Paclitaxel 200 mg/m²	3	66% received chemo, 61% 3 cycles	–	0.5%

Induction						
Rosell et al., 1999	Cis 50 mg/m²/q3w	Ifosfamide 3 g/m² / Mitomycin 6 mg/m²	3	100% received 3 cycles	100%	0%
Roth et al., 1998	Cis 100 mg/m² q4w	Cyclophosphamide 500 mg/m² Etoposide 100 mg/m²/d x3	3 (+3 if ORR)		0%	0%
Depierre et al., 2002	Cis 30 mg/m²/ j x3j	Ifosfamide 1.5 g/m²/d x 3j + Mitomycin 6 mg/m²	2 (+2 if ORR)	90% received 2 cycles (84% PO)	30%	1%
LU22 (Gilligan et al., 2007)	Cis 50 mg/m² q3w / Cis 50 mg/m² q3w / Cis 80 mg/m² q3w / Cis 80 mg/m² q3w / Cb AUC5 / Cb AUC6	Ifosfamide 3 g/m² / Mitomycin 8 mg/m² / Vinblastine 6 mg/m² / Mitomycin 8 mg/m² / Vinorelbine 30 mg/m² d1, d8 / Gemcitabine 1 250 mg/m² d1, d8 / Paclitaxel 175 mg/m² / Docetaxel 75 mg/m²	3	75% received 3 cycles	49%	0%
NATCH (Massuti et al., 2009)	Cb AUC6	Paclitaxel 200 mg/m²	3	97% received chemo, 90% 3 cycles	–	0.5%
Ch.E.S.T. (Scagliotti et al., 2008)	Cis 75 mg/m² q3w	Gemcitabine 1250 mg/m² d1, d8	3	86% received 3 cycles	35%	–

Abbreviations: Cis, cisplatin; Cb, carboplatin; ALPI, Adjuvant Lung Project Italy; IALT, International Adjuvant Lung Trial; BR10: from NCIC-CTG, National Institute of Canada Clinical Trials Group; CALGB, Cancer and Leukemia Group B; ANITA, Adjuvant Navelbine International Trialist Association; * weekly then modified; RT, radiotherapy; PO : post-operative adjuvant setting. The activity of 2 years of adjuvant gefitinib (250 mg/day) or erlotinib (150 mg/d) have been investigated in the National Cancer Institute of Canada BR.19 trial (prematurely closed to accrual) and the RADIANT (Randomized Double-blind Trial in Adjuvant NSCLC with Tarceva) study (presently accruing), respectively. There was no biological selection in BR.19 whereas only patients with immunohistochemically EGFR-positive tumours are included in RADIANT. The IFCT-0801TASTE (Tailored post-Surgical Therapy in Early stage NSCLC) study is evaluating the value of a therapeutic strategy that takes into account the presence of EGFR-activating mutations in surgically resected nonsquamous stage II–IIIA non-N2 NSCLC patients. The patients in the experimental arm receive erlotinib for 1 year if EGFR mutations are present, whereas those individuals with wild type EGFR tumours are evaluated for ERCC1 expression (see below). The use of the anti–vascular endothelial growth factor (VEGF) antibody bevacizumab (15 mg/kg every 3 weeks for 1 year) in association with three different chemotherapy regimens involving cisplatin is also currently being tested in the adjuvant setting (ECOG 1505 trial). The oral antiangiogenic agent pazopanib has been evaluated in the preoperative setting without any postoperative increase in complications. Tumour size was reduced in 87% of patients after a median treatment duration of 18 days. A randomized Phase II/III trial of adjuvant pazopanib versus placebo is ongoing in stage I NSCLC patients (study IFCT 0703).

Multiple biomarkers have been tested to identify subgroups of patients for whom adjuvant treatment would be particularly beneficial. There has been substantial work conducted recently on mechanisms of resistance to chemotherapy. DNA repair components, such as the nucleotide excision repair system, have been the focus of much attention. One of the first biomarkers tested in clinical trials was the excision repair cross-complementation group 1 (ERCC1) enzyme that recognizes and eliminates cisplatin-induced DNA adducts. ERCC1 protein expression (based on immunohistochemistry) was studied in 761 tumours of the IALT trial. The OS of patients with ERCC1-negative tumours (56% of the cases) was significantly prolonged by cisplatin-based chemotherapy (HR 0.65, 95% CI 0.50–0.86, P = 0.002) whereas for patients with ERCC1-positive tumours, adjuvant chemotherapy had no effect (HR 1.14, 95% CI 0.84–1.55, P = 0.40). The value of ERCC-1 is now being tested prospectively in the TASTE trial. In patients with p27Kip1-negative tumours, cisplatin-based chemotherapy showed a trend to prolong survival as compared with surgery alone (HR 0.66, 95% CI 0.50–1.45, P = 0.006, test for interaction = 0.02), whereas OS was not influenced by chemotherapy in p27Kip1-positive tumours. The efficacy of gemcitabine may be related to RRM1 expression (encoding the regulatory subunit of ribonucleotide reductase, a molecular target of gemcitabine), and

RRM1 expression has been suggested to have prognostic value in resected early NSCLC stages. Similarly, the benefit of taxanes has been linked to beta-tubulin mutations. Class III beta tubulin (bTubIII) expression was assessed in 265 of the 482 patients of the JBR.10 trial: high bTubIII expression had a negative prognostic value, but in these patients adjuvant chemotherapy seemed to overcome this effect. A retrospective study has reported a prognostic value of assaying mRNA BRCA1, and this biomarker is currently being evaluated in the adjuvant setting. Few predictive factors have been indentified for UFT although EGFR (epidermal growth factor receptor) mutations may select a sensitive group of patients.

3.8 Conclusions

Meta-analyses have revealed similar HR values for risk of death associated with neoadjuvant or adjuvant therapy: 0.87 (0.81–0.93) for the adjuvant IPD IGR-MRC meta-analysis, 0.89 (0.82–0.96) for the adjuvant IPD LACE pooled analysis, and 0.88 (0.76–1.01) for the more recent non-IPD meta-analysis of neoadjuvant chemotherapy. Nevertheless larger trials and more definitive data, in terms of efficacy and tolerance, support the use of adjuvant chemotherapy. The weak benefit and significant toxicities of cisplatinum based therapy fostered the development of molecular-based therapeutic strategies but this approach remains in the clinical research area.

References

Ardizzoni A., Tiseo M., Boni L., et al. (2006) CISCA (cisplatin vs. carboplatin) meta-analysis: An individual patient data meta-analysis comparing cisplatin versus carboplatin-based chemotherapy in first-line treatment of advanced non-small cell lung cancer (NSCLC). *J Clin Oncol* (Meeting Abstracts) **24**: 7011.

Arriagada R., Dunant A., Pignon J.P., et al. (2009) Long-term results of the international adjuvant lung cancer trial evaluating adjuvant cisplatin-based chemotherapy in resected lung cancer. *J Clin Oncol* **28**: 35–42.

Berghmans T., Paesmans M., Meert A.P., et al. (2005) Survival improvement in resectable non-small cell lung cancer with (neo)adjuvant chemotherapy: results of a meta-analysis of the literature. *Lung Cancer* **49**: 13–23.

Burdett S., Stewart L.A., Rydzewska L (2006) A systematic review and meta-analysis of the literature: chemotherapy and surgery versus surgery alone in non-small cell lung cancer. *J Thorac Oncol* **1**: 611–21.

Butts C.A., Ding K., Seymour L., et al. (2010) Randomized phase III trial of vinorelbine plus cisplatin compared with observation in completely resected stage IB and II non-small-cell lung cancer: updated survival analysis of JBR-10. *J Clin Oncol* **28**: 29–34.

Depierre A., Milleron B., Moro-Sibilot D., *et al.* (2002) Preoperative chemotherapy followed by surgery compared with primary surgery in resectable stage I (except T1N0), II, and IIIa non-small-cell lung cancer. *J Clin Oncol* **20**: 247–53.

Douillard J.Y., Rosell R., De Lena M., *et al.* (2006) Adjuvant vinorelbine plus cisplatin versus observation in patients with completely resected stage IB–IIIA non-small-cell lung cancer (Adjuvant Navelbine International Trialist Association [ANITA]): a randomised controlled trial. *Lancet Oncol* **7**: 719–27.

Fruh M., Rolland E., Pignon J.P., *et al.* (2008) Pooled analysis of the effect of age on adjuvant cisplatin-based chemotherapy for completely resected non-small-cell lung cancer. *J Clin Oncol* **26**: 3573–81.

Gilligan D., Nicolson M., Smith I., *et al.* (2007) Preoperative chemotherapy in patients with resectable non-small cell lung cancer: results of the MRC LU22/NVALT 2/EORTC 08012 multicentre randomised trial and update of systematic review. *Lancet* **369**:1929–37.

Goldstraw P., Crowley J., Chansky K., *et al.* (2007) The IASLC Lung Cancer Staging Project: proposals for the revision of the TNM stage groupings in the forthcoming (seventh) edition of the TNM Classification of malignant tumours. *J Thorac Oncol* **2**: 706–14.

Hamada C., Tanaka F., Ohta M., *et al.* (2005) Meta-analysis of postoperative adjuvant chemotherapy with tegafur-uracil in non-small-cell lung cancer. *J Clin Oncol* **23**: 4999–5006.

Massuti B., Sanchez J.M., Alonso G., *et al.* (2009) Assessing the value of preoperative chemotherapy in early-stage non-small cell lung cancer: mature data and prognostic factors analysis of a Phase III randomized trial of surgery alone vs preoperative Paclitaxel/Carboplatin (PC) vs post-operative PC. Final NATCH data. A Spanish Lung Cancer Group Trial. *Eur J Cancer* **7**: 12.

Olaussen K.A., Dunant A., Fouret P., *et al.* (2006) DNA repair by ERCC1 in non-small-cell lung cancer and cisplatin-based adjuvant chemotherapy. *N Engl J Med* **355**: 983–91.

Pignon J.P., Tribodet H., Scagliotti G.V., *et al.* (2008) Lung adjuvant cisplatin evaluation: a pooled analysis by the LACE Collaborative Group. *J Clin Oncol* **26**: 3552–9.

Rosell R., Gomez-Codina J., Camps C., *et al.* (1999) Preresectional chemotherapy in stage IIIA non-small-cell lung cancer: a 7-year assessment of a randomized controlled trial. *Lung Cancer* **26**: 7–14.

Roth J.A., Atkinson E.N., Fossella F., *et al.* (1998) Long-term follow-up of patients enrolled in a randomized trial comparing perioperative chemotherapy and surgery with surgery alone in resectable stage IIIA non-small-cell lung cancer. *Lung Cancer* **21**: 1–6.

Scagliotti G.V., Fossati R., Torri V., *et al.* (2003) Randomized study of adjuvant chemotherapy for completely resected stage I, II, or IIIA non-small-cell lung cancer. *J Natl Cancer Inst* **95**: 1453–61.

Scagliotti G.V., Pastorino U., Vansteenkiste J.F., et al. (2008) A phase III randomized study of surgery alone or surgery plus preoperative gemcitabine-cisplatin in early-stage non-small cell lung cancer (NSCLC): Follow-up data of Ch.E.S. J Clin Oncol (Meeting Abstracts) 26: 7508.

Stewart L.A., Burdett S., Tierney J.F., et al. (2007) on behalf of the NSCLC Collaborative Group: Surgery and adjuvant chemotherapy (CT) compared to surgery alone in non-small cell lung cancer (NSCLC): A meta-analysis using individual patient data (IPD) from randomized clinical trials (RCT). J Clin Oncol (Meeting Abstracts) 25: 7552.

Strauss G.M., Herndon J.E., II, Maddaus M.A., et al. (2008) Adjuvant paclitaxel plus carboplatin compared with observation in stage IB non-small-cell lung cancer: CALGB 9633 with the Cancer and Leukemia Group B, Radiation Therapy Oncology Group, and North Central Cancer Treatment Group Study Groups. J Clin Oncol 26: 5043–51.

Strauss G.M., Herndon J., Maddaus M.A., et al. (2004) Randomized clinical trial of adjuvant chemotherapy with paclitaxel and carboplatin following resection in stage IB non-small cell lung cancer (NSCLC): Report of Cancer and Leukemia Group B (CALGB) Protocol 9633. J Clin Oncol (Meeting Abstracts) 22: 7019.

Suehisa H., Toyooka S., Hotta K., et al. (2007) Epidermal growth factor receptor mutation status and adjuvant chemotherapy with uracil-tegafur for adenocarcinoma of the lung. J Clin Oncol 25: 3952–7.

Waller D., Peake M.D., Stephens R.J., et al. (2004) Chemotherapy for patients with non-small cell lung cancer: the surgical setting of the Big Lung Trial. Eur J Cardiothorac Surg 26: 173–82.

Westeel V., Milleron B., Quoix E., et al. (2009) Results of the IFCT 0002 phase III study comparing a preoperative and a perioperative chemotherapy (CT) with two different CT regimens in resectable non-small cell lung cancer (NSCLC). J Clin Oncol (Meeting Abstracts) 27: 7530.

Chapter 4

Combined modality therapy for locally advanced NSCLC

Margaret Edwards and Hak Choy

Key points

- Multiple clinical trials have shown improved survival when combining chemotherapy with thoracic radiation therapy for definitive treatment of locally advanced NSCLC
- Up-front concurrent chemoradiation therapy provides the best treatment outcomes when compared with sequential therapy or induction chemotherapy, although the efficacy of concurrent chemoradiation must be balanced with its increased toxicity
- The benefit of 'consolidation' chemotherapy is not supported by phase III clinical trials when full dose chemotherapy is given during the concurrent phase
- While a 'platinum doublet' is the most commonly used chemotherapy regimen with concurrent thoracic radiation therapy, the optimal chemotherapy agents remain controversial
- Targeted biologic agents have shown promise in treatment and will likely have an increasing future role
- New technological developments in radiation therapy, such as image-guidance, allow more precise targeting of tumour with increasing radiotherapy dose and normal tissue sparing, thus increasing the rate of local control.

4.1 **Introduction**

The majority of non-small-cell lung cancers are not diagnosed at an early stage that can be surgically resected with a curative intent. While some patients have extrathoracic metastatic disease at diagnosis, 30 to 40% of non-small-cell lung cancer cases present with locally advanced disease, which is disease confined to the thorax with a potential for cure with combined modality therapy. Locally advanced disease involves the ipsilateral mediastinal lymph nodes (American Joint Committee on Cancer [AJCC] 6th Edition Tl-3 N2 MO, Stage IIIA) or contralateral mediastinal or hilar, or any scalene or supraclavicular lymph nodes (AJCC 6th Edition Tl-2 N3 MO, Stage IIIB), without evidence of extrathoracic metastases. Patients with a centrally located primary tumour involving mediastinal structures (AJCC 6th Edition T4 Nx MO, Stage IIIB) are also considered to have locally advanced disease that is not traditionally treated with surgical resection. The presence of a malignant pleural effusion places a patient in a category know as 'wet IIIB' which is more appropriately treated as a metastatic or stage IV NSCLC.

4.2 **Combined chemotherapy and radiation therapy**

Radiation therapy plays an essential role in definitive treatment of locally advanced NSCLC. Although historical survival rates using radiation therapy alone for locally advanced NSCLC are poor, treatment with chemotherapy alone also produces inferior outcomes compared with combined modality therapy. A phase III study by Kubota *et.al.* treated stage III NSCLC patients with 1 of 3 regimens of platinum-based chemotherapy followed by randomization, if the patient had not progressed, to observation or 50 to 70 Gy of thoracic radiation therapy. This trial showed a benefit to including radiation therapy as part of treatment, with an increase in the survival rate from 9% to 36% at 2 years and 3% to 29% at 3 years with the addition of radiation therapy (see Table 4.1).

4.3 **Sequential chemotherapy and radiation therapy**

Sequential chemotherapy followed by radiation therapy allows delivery of full doses of both chemotherapy and radiation therapy, with the rationale that chemotherapy can target any micrometastatic disease while thoracic radiation can control disease in the chest. The change in standard of care to combined chemotherapy

Table 4.1 Selected multicenter randomized trials of locally advanced NSCLC

Study	Sequence	Pt #	RT Dose (Gy)	Chemo	Median survival (months)	Overall survival 3 yr (%)	Overall survival 5 yr (%)	Acute ≥grade 3 esophagitis (%)
Kubota	CT	32	50–70	MVP	14.9	3	–	–
	CT→RT	31		MVP	15.4	29		
CALGB 8433	RT	77	60	–	9.6	6	6	–
	CT→RT	78	60	Cddp/vinblastine	13.7	24	17	
West Japan Lung Cancer Group (Furuse)	CT→RT	158	56	MVP	13.3	15	9	2
	ChemoRT (split course)	156	56 (split course)	MVP	16.5	22	16	3
RTOG 9410	CT→RT	201	60	Cddp/vinblastine	14.6	–	10	4
	ChemoRT	201	60	Cddp/vinblastine	17		16	23
	ChemoRT (bid)	193	69.6 (bid)	Cddp/etoposide	15.1		13	46
LAMP (Belani)	CT→RT	91	63	Carbo/taxol	13.0	17	–	3
	CT→ChemoRT	74	63	Carbo/taxol → low dose carbo/taxol	12.7	15		19
	ChemoRT→CT	92	63	low dose carbo/taxol → carbo/taxol	16.3	17		28

Table 4.1 (Contd.)

Study	Sequence	Pt #	RT Dose (Gy)	Chemo	Median survival (months)	Overall survival 3 yr (%)	Overall survival 5 yr (%)	Acute ≥grade 3 esophagitis (%)
HOG (Hanna)	ChemoRT	74	59.4	Cddp/etoposide	23.2	26.1	–	17.2
	ChemoRT|CT	73	59.4	Cddp/etoposide → docetaxel	21.2	27.1		17.2
SWOG 0023	ChemoRT → CT → gefitinib	118	61	Cddp/etoposide → docetaxel → gefitinib	23*	–	–	13
	ChemoRT → CT → placebo	125	61	Cddp/etoposide → docetaxel → placebo	35*			
Yuan	ChemoRT (ENI)	100	60–64 (ENI)	Cddp/etoposide	15	–	18.3	5
	ChemoRT (IF)	100	68–74 (IF)	Cddp/etoposide	20		25.1	4

Pt # = number of patients ; RT = radiotherapy; CT = chemotherapy; bid = twice daily; MVP = mitomycin, vindesine, cisplatin; carbo/taxol = carboplatin/taxol; cddp = cisplatin; ENI = elective nodal irradiation; IF = involved field irradiation

* Of 571 eligible patients, survival only reflects the 243 that had not progressed after chemoRT → chemo and were randomized to gefitinib or placebo

and radiotherapy for locally advanced NSCLC occurred in the 1990s, based on multiple clinical trials. In CALGB 8433, median survival improved from 9.6 to 13.7 months with the addition of induction chemotherapy with cisplatin and vinblastine prior to 60 Gy of thoracic radiation therapy. In the 155 randomized patients, the 5-year survival rate tripled, from 6 to 17%, with combined chemotherapy and radiation therapy over radiation therapy alone. Several other large randomized trials confirmed the benefit of a combination of sequential chemotherapy and radiation therapy.

4.4 **Concurrent chemoradiation**

With concurrent chemoradiation therapy, chemotherapy can also act as a radiosensitizer for tumours in the chest by inhibiting repair of radiation-induced damage, decreasing tumour cell repopulation between fractions of radiation therapy, or enhancing killing of radio-resistant clones. An early trial comparing concurrent chemoradiation therapy with sequential therapy was conducted by the West Japan Lung Cancer Group, enrolling 314 patients. Both treatment arms received chemotherapy consisting of mitomycin, vindesine and cisplatin. The concurrent arm was treated with 56 Gy of split course radiation therapy, while the sequential arm was treated with continuous radiation therapy to a dose of 56 Gy. Concurrent chemoradiation therapy improved the response rate from 66% to 84% and the median survival from 13.3 to 16.5 months when compared with sequential therapy. This improved outcome was achieved in spite of the split course radiotherapy in the concurrent arm, which is considered to be an inferior method of treatment. RTOG 9410 was a 610-patient phase III clinical trial for inoperable stage II and III NSCLC that showed the best outcome with concurrent chemotherapy and daily radiation therapy, when compared to sequential chemotherapy followed by radiation therapy. The chemotherapy given in these 2 arms of the trial were cisplatin and vinblastine. Median survival was 17 months with concurrent chemotherapy and daily radiation therapy versus 14.6 months with sequential therapy. RTOG 9410 also sought to test the benefit of hyperfractionated (twice-daily) radiation therapy by including a third arm in the trial of concurrent cisplatin, etoposide, and twice daily radiation therapy. This treatment group did not demonstrate improved outcomes over the sequential therapy group, possibly due to increased toxicity with hyperfractionated radiation therapy. The concurrent chemoradiation therapy arm with daily radiotherapy in RTOG 94-10 also reported higher rates of acute grade 3–4 non-hematologic toxicity, including esophagitis, compared with the sequential chemoradiation therapy arm. Concurrent chemo-radiation therapy with a third generation agent, such as paclitaxel has been widely used due to the favourable toxicity profile. The goal of additional tumour cell killing with concurrent chemoradiation therapy must be balanced with the possible increased risk of normal tissue toxicity, including myelosuppression or non-hematologic toxicity such as esophagitis or pneumonitis.

4.5 Consolidation chemotherapy

Other options for the sequencing of chemotherapy and radiation therapy are diagrammed in Figure 4.1. Additional chemotherapy with docetaxel after definitive chemoradiation, known as consolidation therapy, has been a schema with some popularity based on positive results in phase II clinical trials. However, a randomized phase III trial by the Hoosier Oncology Group did not provide support for the benefit of consolidation chemotherapy when full dose cisplatin and etoposide are given during the concurrent phase. The trial attempted to show improved survival by giving three cycles of docetaxel after concurrent full dose cisplatin, etoposide, and thoracic radiation therapy to 59.4 Gy. The trial was closed after analyzing the initial 203 enrolled patients and determining that there was no survival difference between the concurrent chemoradiation therapy followed by observation (median 23.2 months) versus the arm receiving consolidation docetaxel (median 21.2 months). Docetaxel consolidation was also associated with higher rates of hospitalization, grade 3/4 toxicities, and treatment-related deaths. The lack of benefit with consolidative chemotherapy seen in this trial may be due to the particular agent chosen or perhaps the use of a single agent rather than a platinum doublet. Typically around 4 cycles of chemotherapy are given for almost all other stages of lung cancer. Consolidation with chemotherapy or a targeted agent may still play an important role in the future for this patient population. Meanwhile, consolidation chemotherapy is an important part of treatment when low dose weekly chemotherapy is administered during the concurrent phase of treatment.

4.6 Optimal chemotherapy

A variety of chemotherapy regimens have been tested with concurrent radiation therapy for locally advanced NSCLC. There is little data to declare one of them as standard of care. Randomized comparisons of various chemotherapy combinations for metastatic NSCLC have been done, and their results are often extrapolated to locally advanced NSCLC. A 'platinum doublet', meaning cisplatin or carboplatin plus another drug, is the most commonly delivered regimen. Choice of a particular regimen is often based on side effect profiles, availability factors, or ease of administration.

4.7 Targeted combined modality therapy

Increased understanding of molecular pathways involved in tumour growth and progression has given rise to a new era of targeted biologic agents. The theoretical advantage of targeted therapy is its greater effect on tumour cells than normal tissue. Since lung tumours are genetically heterogeneous and can demonstrate several mechanisms of resistance in response to biologic agents, the best improvement in outcomes for locally advanced NSCLC with targeted therapy will likely be seen in combination with chemotherapy and radiation therapy.

Both small molecule enzyme inhibitors and antibodies have been developed that target important signal transduction pathways. Epidermal growth factor receptor (EGFR) tyrosine kinase inhibitors, such as gefitinib and erlotinib, have shown activity in subsets of patients with advanced NSCLC, but experience with radiotherapy is limited. SWOG 0023 attempted to improve survival in inoperable stage III NSCLC by adding maintenance gefitinib if patients had not progressed after concurrent chemoradiation therapy and docetaxel consolidation. However, there was no benefit to maintenance gefitinib, with a median survival time of 23 months in the gefitinib arm versus 35 months for the placebo arm.

The chimeric antibody to EGFR, cetuximab, was used in locally advanced NSCLC in an RTOG phase II trial confirming the feasibility of delivering concurrent cetuximab with standard chemoradiation therapy. One of the aims of an ongoing phase III RTOG trial is to demonstrate a survival benefit to the addition of cetuximab to concurrent chemoradiation therapy for locally advanced NSCLC.

Many other targeted agents are being evaluated in advanced disease and will likely also be combined with radiotherapy in locally advanced NSCLC.

4.8 Optimizing radiation therapy

We cannot improve overall survival and quality of life for locally advanced NSCLC (LANSCLC) patients without improving local control. Thus, efforts to increase local control by improving radiation therapy techniques remain a key strategy in LANSCLC. Impressive progress in technology has changed the delivery of radiation therapy to allow more precise targeting of tumour and avoidance of normal structures for the last decade. 3D conformal radiotherapy (3-DCRT) and intensity modulated radiation therapy (IMRT), based on computed tomography (CT) planning, are possible due to modern computer and software advances. Other technologies crucial in radiation therapy for lung tumours include imaging that characterizes organ motion with respiration (see Figure 4.2) and positron emission tomography (PET), to better delineate tumour versus other lung pathology. All of these have allowed reduction of treatment volumes and dose escalation of fractionated radiotherapy.

4.9 **Radiation therapy dose and volume**

55 to 64 Gy has been the dose of radiotherapy traditionally given for locally advanced NSCLC over the past 30 years. These typical doses were established in the era prior to CT planning and other technology that allows more precise tumour targeting. In addition, the traditional treatment field for locally advanced NSCLC included elective nodal irradiation of the mediastinal and, if an upper lobe lesion, then ipsilateral supraclavicular lymph node regions, due to concern for recurrence in the next echelon of lymph nodes. This larger field size limits the dose that can be safely delivered without excessive toxicity. While still controversial, many clinicians now only irradiate the gross disease as defined by biopsy or imaging modalites such as CT or PET (see Figure 4.3). There are several reasons for this shift in treatment strategy. One is evidence that local failures within the treatment volume at a dose around 60 Gy are common, so efforts at eradicating the primary tumour and involved lymph nodes seem most crucial. A second reason is that isolated failure in an initially uninvolved lymph node area is rare. A trial by Yuan et.al. randomized 200 patients with stage III NSCLC to involved-field irradiation to 68 to 74 Gy versus elective nodal irradiation to a dose of 60 to 64 Gy in combination with concurrent cisplatin-based chemotherapy. The involved-field irradiation group had a higher overall response rate, 90% vs. 79%, and better 5-year rate local control, 51% vs. 36%. Toxicity was not significantly different between the two arms, except for less pneumonitis in the involved-field irradiation arm, suggesting that treating a smaller field to a higher dose is the better overall treatment.

Recent phase I and II trials have demonstrated the feasibility of delivering doses higher than 60 Gy with concurrent weekly low dose chemotherapy and suggested a possible increase in median survival with a more potent dose. Several cooperative group trials and University of North Carolina studies had promising results when escalating dose to 74 Gy. An ongoing randomized phase III RTOG trial seeks confirm the results of nonrandomized trials of dose escalation and to establish the efficacy of a dose of 74 Gy with concurrent weekly low dose chemotherapy followed two cycles of full dose consolidative chemotherapy for LANSCLC.

4.10 Image-guided radiation therapy

Recently, there has been increasing use of image-guided radiation therapy (IGRT) to improve the accuracy of dose delivery. IGRT involves frequent imaging to account for change in location of a tumour between fractions of radiation therapy (interfraction motion) and sometimes motion of the tumour with respiration during delivery of a fraction of radiation therapy (intrafraction motion). IGRT includes modalities such as daily ultrasound, kilovoltage (kV) imaging such as x-rays or kV cone beam CT, or megavoltage (MV) imaging such as helical MV CT or MV cone beam CT. Adaptive radiotherapy is the concept of using frequent imaging to alter treatment based on changes in the tumour or normal tissue during the course of treatment. This can be important in treatment of NSCLC since tumours can shrink considerably during treatment, allowing greater avoidance of normal structures when the treatment plan is modified. For example, three weeks into a 7-week course of thoracic radiation therapy, a new planning CT scan may show significant reduction in tumour size. At that point, a new treatment plan can be created that reduces the dose given to normal lung tissue and thus decreases the risk of pneumonitis and long-term fibrosis.

4.11 Conclusion

Over the past 30 years, numerous incremental advances in locally advanced NSCLC treatment have translated into a survival increase of about a year, as median survival in randomized phase III trials has risen from less than 1 year to almost 2 years. Combined modality therapy with chemotherapy and radiation therapy is the accepted standard for unresectable disease. Molecular targeted therapy may play an increasing role in the future, together with further refinement in radiation therapy delivery techniques. There are still many new treatment modalities to explore and much progress needed in finding a cure for locally advanced NSCLC.

Further reading

Belani C.P., Choy H., Bonomi P., et al. (2005) Combined chemoradiotherapy regimens of paclitaxel and carboplatin for locally advanced non-small-cell lung cancer: a randomized phase II locally advanced multi-modality protocol J Clin Oncol **23**(25): 5883–91.

Curran, W., Scott C.B., Langer C.J., et al. (2003) Long-term benefit is observed in a phase III comparison of sequential vs concurrent chemo-radiation for patients with unresectable NSCLC: RTOG 9410 Proceedings of ASCO **22**: 621a.

Dillman R.O., Herndon J., Seagren S.L., *et al.* (1996) Improved survival in stage III non-small-cell lung cancer: seven-year follow-up of cancer and leukemia group B (CALGB) 8433 trial *J Natl Cancer Inst* **88**(17): 1210–5.

Furuse K., Fukuoka M., Kawahara M., *et al.* (1999) Phase III study of concurrent versus sequential thoracic radiotherapy in combination with mitomycin, vindesine, and cisplatin in unresectable stage III non-small-cell lung cancer *J Clin Oncol* **17**(9): 2692–9.

Hanna N., Neubauer M., Yiannoutsos C., *et al.* (2008) Phase III study of cisplatin, etoposide, and concurrent chest radiation with or without consolidation docetaxel in patients with inoperable stage III non-small-cell lung cancer: the Hoosier Oncology Group and U.S. Oncology *J Clin Oncol* **26**(35): 5755–60.

Kelly K., Chansky K., Gaspar L.E., *et al.* (2008) Phase III trial of maintenance gefitinib or placebo after concurrent chemoradiotherapy and docetaxel consolidation in inoperable stage III non-small-cell lung cancer: SWOG S0023 *J Clin Oncol* **26**(15): 2450–56.

Kubota K., Furuse K., Kawahara M., *et al.* (1994) Role of radiotherapy in combined modality treatment of locally advanced non-small-cell lung cancer *J Clin Oncol* **12**(8): 1547–52.

Lee C.B., Stinchcombe T.E., Moore D.T., *et al.* (2009) Late complications of high-dose (>/=66 Gy) thoracic conformal radiation therapy in combined modality trials in unresectable stage III non-small cell lung cancer *J Thorac Oncol* **4**(1): 74–9.

Yuan S., Sun X., Li M., *et al.* (2007) A randomized study of involved-field irradiation versus elective nodal irradiation in combination with concurrent chemotherapy for inoperable stage III nonsmall cell lung cancer *Am J Clin Oncol* **30**(3): 239–44.

Chapter 5

Systemic therapy for advanced NSCLC, efficacy, and toxicity

Taylor M. Ortiz and Pasi A. Jänne

Key points

- Palliate symptoms first.
- Chemotherapy improves survival over best supportive care.
- Some oligometastatic NSCLC is appropriate for aggressive treatment with curative intent.
- Personalized therapy based on *EGFR* mutation status can improve progression free survival and avoid ineffective therapies.
- Tailoring biologic and chemotherapies based on tumor histology can maximize treatment efficacy.

5.1 Introduction

At the time of presentation, more than 50% of patients with lung cancer will present with advanced disease (Jemal et al., 2009). Of those who present with resectable disease, 41% of these patients develop a recurrence (Sugimura et al., 2007). Given these sobering statistics, a treating physicians' primary charge in the care of lung cancer patients is the care of patients with advanced disease. In this chapter, the appropriate care of patients with advanced disease is discussed, including results of new studies that help providers select therapies based on genetic and histologic characteristics.

5.2 Palliate symptoms first

With the rare exception of oligometastatic disease, advanced NSCLC is largely not a curable illness; therefore, one of the primary goals of treatment should be the appropriate palliation of the symptoms of lung cancer with attention to quality of life.

From the time of diagnosis of advanced disease, providers should clearly relate the goals of care to patients in order to set appropriate expectations for patients and family (Gabrijel *et al.*, 2008). Along these lines, careful and continuous attention to symptom management needs to be chief among the goals of patients, family, and providers (see Chapter 7, Palliative Therapy in NSCLC). Local therapy for symptomatic disease is an important part of appropriate palliative care and is covered in detail in Chapter 8.

5.3 Chemotherapy versus best supportive care

For several years the benefit of chemotherapy for metastatic disease was in question. To evaluate the utility of chemotherapy for advanced NSCLC, several studies were conducted to compare systemic chemotherapy to best supportive care. The largest of these studies randomized patients with NSCLC that were not eligible for surgical resection to receive either best supportive care or best supportive care plus one of four cisplatin-based combination chemotherapies (Spiro *et al.*, 2004). The median age of the patients in this study was 65, and 22% had a WHO PS of 2–3. In this cohort of 725 subjects, the patients assigned to receive chemotherapy lived longer than those assigned to best supportive care alone, with a median overall survival of 8.0 months versus 5.7 months (p = .0006). This benefit appears to have occurred without any significant detriment to quality of life based on pre-defined criteria; however, quality of life data was only determined in patients from two centres and in less than 40% of the total patients on study.

These results confirmed the findings of a 1995 meta-analysis of 1,190 patients with advanced NSCLC receiving platinum-based therapies that showed a 10% improvement in survival at one year in patients treated with chemotherapy plus best supportive care versus best supportive care alone (HR for death 0.73, P<0.0001). A 2008 update of this meta-analysis reviewing the outcome of 2,714 patients randomized to chemotherapy versus BSC confirmed these benefits, with a HR of 0.77 for patients assigned to chemotherapy (p< = .0001).

Despite the demonstrated benefits in overall survival, some patients may choose not to pursue chemotherapy for advanced disease; in that case, aggressive supportive care measures conducted in a team based approach should to be an important part of patient care (see Palliative Care).

5.4 Personalizing care of patients with advanced NSCLC

With data confirming a benefit to chemotherapy for advanced lung cancer, a great deal of research has gone into determining which chemotherapy regimen offers the best survival, and whether personalizing therapy based on tumour characteristics may improve the outcome. In the past, the treatment of advanced NSCLC was more generally applied to all patients without alteration for histologic or molecular subtypes of disease. As new chemotherapeutics, biologics, and targeted agents have been developed, studies have shown that subtypes of NSCLC may respond to therapy differently. In many cases, the difference in response is well understood molecularly, and in the future, the hope is that therapies will be delivered with much more molecular rationale, sparing patients from treatments to which their tumour will be refractory and maximizing the utility of potentially beneficial therapies.

5.5 The exception for oligometastatic NSCLC

Oligometastatic lung cancer, when disease is limited to a localized site in the chest with otherwise a single metastatic site in either an adrenal gland or in the brain, can sometimes be an exception to the typically incurable nature of stage IV NSCLC. Although this group is a small fraction of patients with metastatic disease, there is a subset of patients in this group that make up much of the 'tail of the curve' in studies of patients with stage IV disease and can become long-term survivors. Therefore, providers must ensure that there is a careful, multidisciplinary evaluation of these patients for whom a cure is possible. Those with solitary sites outside the chest not in the adrenal gland or brain (i.e. liver or bone) are considered by most to be rarely cured with aggressive therapy.

Successful treatment of adrenal metastases from NSCLC with long term survival was first documented in 2 patients treated with adrenalectomy and definitive local therapy to the primary lung lesions, with these two patients surviving 5 years and 13 years from adrenalectomy (Twomey et al., 1982). Efforts have been made to better clarify the prognostic importance of synchronous versus metachronous adrenal metastases in patients with NSCLC, defined as occurring within or beyond six months of primary tumour diagnosis, respectively. Tanvetyanon and colleagues published a systematic review of the outcomes for synchronous and metachronous adrenal metastases in 114 patients with NSCLC, culling data from 10 studies published between 1990 and 2007 (Tanvetyanon et al., 2008). The median survival of patients with isolated synchronous adrenal metastases in this study was 12 months versus 31 months for patients with metachronous lesions; however, regardless of the disease free interval, the synchronous and the metachronous cohorts had a 5-year survival of 26% and 25%, respectively, indicating that a substantial portion of patients with either synchronous or metachronous adrenal metastases may be long-term survivors with aggressive adrenal and thoracic therapy.

Several studies have been published on the successful long-term outcomes of patients with NSCLC with a solitary brain metastasis with 5-year survival ranging between 7 and 21% (Billing et al., 2001; Hu et al., 2006; Flannery et al., 2008). Hu and colleagues published findings of a retrospective cohort of 84 patients treated for NSCLC who initially presented with a concurrent single brain metastasis, finding that the vast majority of the long-term survivors were those with thoracic AJCC stage I disease in addition to the single brain metastasis, with median survival of the thoracic stage I patients that received definitive therapy of 25.6 months (Hu et al., 2006). Another retrospective study of 42 patients suggests that for patients with good performance status and able to undergo definitive therapy of thoracic disease in addition to the single brain metastasis, long term survival can be achieved, with 5-year median overall survival of 21% (Flannery et al., 2008). Although these studies are limited by their retrospective nature and small size, for patients with early stage thoracic disease, a good performance status, and a solitary brain metastasis, long-term survival is possible in patients with aggressive treatment. It also implies that for patients with more advanced intra-thoracic disease, long-term survival is exceedingly rare.

5.6 Personalizing treatments for advanced NSCLC

5.6.1 EGFR mutations and EGFR tyrosine kinase inhibitors

Early interest in EGFR as a target in lung cancer due to its activation in malignancies and its status as a 'druggable' target (a receptor tyrosine kinase) brought studies of two small-molecule tyrosine kinase inhibitors, gefitinib (Iressa®, AstraZeneca) and erlotinib (Tarceva®, OSI Pharmaceuticals). Initial studies of gefitinib in the second line were promising, and earned accelerated FDA approval; however, in a phase 3 study comparing gefitinib to best supportive care in a non-genotyped population, treatment with gefitinib was not found to be superior to placebo, and FDA approval was withdrawn (Thatcher et al., 2005). Erlotinib later went on to receive approval in the second-line after results of a phase 3 randomized study showed that treatment with erlotinib resulted in a 2-month prolongation in median overall survival versus placebo (6.7 vs 4.7 months) (Shepherd *et al.*, 2005) .

Researchers noted that a subgroup of patients seemed to have particularly vigorous responses to erlotinib, and three groups went on to identify that deletions in exon 19 or missense mutations in exon 21 of *EGFR* predicted for a response to erlotinib or gefitinib (Lynch *et al.*, 2004; Paez *et al.*, 2004; Pao *et al.*, 2004). These mutations, which occur in the kinase domain of *EGFR*, trigger autophosphorylation and downstream activation of the targets of EGFR, causing cell division and resistance to apoptosis. Demographically, patients with *EGFR* mutations tend to be more often females, have adenocarcinoma histology, be of East Asian descent, and lifelong non-smokers.

Given that *EGFR* mutations appeared to predict responses to erlotinib or gefitinib, researchers conducted several phase 2 studies using these drugs as first-line therapy in patients with *EGFR* mutations, showing that there was between a 55 and 75% response rate (Asahinia *et al.*, 2006; Inoue *et al.*, 2006 Sequist *et al.*, 2008). Recently, Mok and colleagues published a phase 3 study randomizing 1217 treatment-naïve, East Asian patients who were non-smokers or former light smokers to either first-line gefitinib or carboplatin and paclitaxel. In a pre-specified subset analysis, patients with *EGFR* activating mutations had an improved progression free survival (PFS) with gefitinib versus chemotherapy (HR for progression or death 0.48, 95% CI, 0.36 to 0.64; P<0.001), and patients without *EGFR* activating mutations had an improved PFS with chemotherapy (hazard ratio for progression or death with gefitinib, 2.85; 95% CI, 2.05 to 3.98; P<0.001) (Mok *et al.*, 2009) . Overall survival in this early analysis, however, was not found to be significantly different for patients with activating *EGFR* mutations.

It is generally felt that in patients with activating *EGFR* mutations, gefitinib and erlotinib are equally effective, but this has not been evaluated in large, prospective studies. Currently, only erlotinib is available in the United States; gefitinib and erlotinib are both available internationally. Toxicities include an acneiform rash (any grade, 60–75%) and diarrhea (any grade, 50–55%) (Shepherd *et al.*, 2005; Sequist *et al.*, 2008).

Combinations employing erlotinib or gefitinib with chemotherapy in unselected patient populations have been largely disappointing (Giaccone *et al.*, 2004; Herbst *et al.*, 2004; Herbst *et al.*, 2005; Gatzmeier *et al.*, 2007); however, studies are ongoing to evaluate this strategy in patients with *EGFR* mutations.

5.6.2 **Angiogenesis inhibitors**

Sustained angiogenesis is a hallmark of cancer, and researchers have designed drugs to target factors important in tumour angiogenesis.

Vascular endothelial growth factor (VEGF) is an endothelial-cell specific mitogen that has been shown to be upregulated in NSCLC (Mattern *et al.*, 1996). In the E4599 study, 878 patients with advanced NSCLC and good performance status were randomized to receive carboplatin plus paclitaxel with or without a humanized monoclonal antibody to VEGF, (bevacizumab, Avastin®, Genentech) (Sandler *et al.*, 2006). Due to concerns for bleeding seen in a previous phase 2 study (Johnson *et al.*, 2004), the study was limited to patients with non-squamous histology, without a history of hemoptysis, no brain metastases, not receiving anticoagulation, and without cavitary lung lesions.

E4599 demonstrated that patients who received bevacizumab had a median survival of 12.3 months versus 10.3 months in patients who did not receive bevacizumab (p = .003). There were distinct toxicities associated with bevacizumab treatment; patients receiving bevacizumab had a higher incidence of pulmonary haemorrhage, hypertension, and proteinuria, and a total of 15 patients in the bevacizumab group died of treatment related toxicities versus 2 in the control arm (p = .001), mainly due to pulmonary hemorrhage and neutropenic fever. Despite these toxicities, there was a persistent benefit in overall survival in the arm randomized to bevacizumab; however, providers must carefully exclude patients with a significant bleeding risk and monitor patients closely during therapy.

A recent study appears to confirm the safety of adding bevacizumab to chemotherapy in patients with non-squamous NSCLC with treated brain metastases, with zero patients of 106 developing CNS hemorrhage at a median follow-up of 6.3 months (Socinski *et al.*, 2009).

5.6.3 Bevacizumab ineligible patients: the importance of histology

Historically, there was no evidence that particular treatments were differentially effective in various NSCLC histologies. However, novel agents and molecular studies have changed the landscape of modern NSCLC therapy, and recent data suggests that personalizing therapy based on the histologic subtype of NSCLC can improve survival.

In a large, phase 3 non-inferiority study, 1,725 chemotherapy-naïve patients with NSCLC were randomized to receive either cisplatin plus pemetrexed or cisplatin plus gemcitabine for 4 cycles. Among all patients, the regimens were found to be non-inferior (median survival 10.3 months in both arms, HR 0.94, CI 0.84 to 1.05); however, in a subgroup analysis based on tumour histology, patients with adenocarcinoma and large-cell carcinoma had superior overall survival with pemetrexed (12.6 vs 10.9 months in patients with adenocarcinoma and 10.4 vs 6.7 months in patients with large-cell carcinoma) compared to patients with squamous histology, who had improved survival with gemcitabine (10.8 vs 9.4 mos) (Scagliotti *et al.*, 2008). This subgroup analysis was not a pre-specified endpoint of the study, but other studies with pemetrexed have also supported its activity in non-squamous histology (Hanna et al., 2004; Scagliotti et al., 2009). A postulated mechanism why patients with squamous histology have an inferior response to pemetrexed is that squamous cell NSCLC tends to have higher expression of thymidilate synthase, the protein that is inhibited by pemetrexed (Ceppi et al., 2006). A phase 3 study is ongoing evaluating whether a combination of carboplatin, pemetrexed, and bevacizumab is superior to carboplatin, paclitaxel, and bevacizumab (Patel et al., 2009).

5.6.4 Non-antibody containing chemotherapies
For patients that are not suitable for triplet therapy using bevacizumab, who do not have activating mutations in EGFR, and are not appropriate for pemetrexed or gemcitabine, a platinum-based doublet is the standard of care. In the TAX326 study, 1,218 patients with advanced NSCLC were randomized to receive either cisplatin and vinorelbine, cisplatin and docetaxel, or carboplatin and docetaxel. The patients treated with docetaxel and cisplatin had a median survival of 11.3 months versus 10.1 months for the group receiving vinorelbine and cisplatin (p = 0.044) with a favourable toxicity profile (Fossella et al., 2003).

5.6.5 EGFR-targeting antibodies
Cetuximab (Erbitux®, ImClone) is a humanized, monoclonal anti-EGFR antibody that is currently FDA approved in colorectal and head and neck cancers. EGFR is expressed in more than 80% of lung cancers, and elevated EGFR expression is associated with a worse outcome (Salomon et al., 1995; Fujino et al., 1996) . For this reason, cetuximab has been evaluated in combination with platinum doublet chemotherapy in the FLEX trial (Pirker et al., 2009). In this study, 1,125 patients with advanced NSCLC and with tumours expressing EGFR were randomized to receive cisplatin, vinorelbine, and cetuximab versus cisplatin and vinorelbine alone. The median overall survival for patients who received cetuximab was 11.3 vs 10.1 months without cetuximab (p = .044), with the primary toxicities being acneiform rash, diarrhoea, and rare infusion reactions. Interestingly, there was no difference in progression free survival between the two groups (the primary endpoint), a finding that has not been fully explained. Given the paucity of data using cetuximab in the first line in lung cancer, and the disparate results of PFS and OS from FLEX, the role of cetuximab in NSCLC is not completely clear.

5.6.6 Duration of therapy
The optimal number of cycles of doublet chemotherapy has not been definitively determined, but studies appear to suggest that 4 cycles is reasonable, and that therapy beyond six cycles may improve

Table 5.1 Select pivotal trials in advanced NSCLC				
Trial	Therapy	Outcome	Benefit	Notes
E4599 (Sandler et al., 2006)	Carboplatin + paclitaxel +/– bevacizumab	Addition of bevacizumab better	12.3 m. vs 10.3 mos median O.S.	Excluded squams, and other bleeding risk. 15 deaths on treatment arm vs. 5
Scagliotti et al., 2008	Cisplatin + pemetrexed vs cisplatin + gemcitabine	Non-inferiority of cisplatin-pemetrexed	10.3 m. O.S. in both arms	Cisplatin + pemetrexed better in non-squamous histology; cisplatin+ gemcitabine better in squamous
IPASS (Mok et al., 2009)	Gefitnib vs carboplatin + paclitaxel	Gefitinib improved PFS in this patient population	HR for progression 0.74	Better outcome for gefitinib for Asian never or former-light smokers with adenocarcinoma. EGFR mutatnts had HR of 0.48
Ciuleanul et al., 2008	Maintenance pemetrexed + BSC vs Placebo + BSC	Maintenance pemetrexed improved O.S.	O.S. 13.4 m. vs 10.6 m.	Only 18% of patients assigned to control arm received pemetrexed after progression

response rate without an improvement in overall survival (Smith et al., 2001; Socinski et al., 2002; von Plessen et al., 2006). Therefore, limiting therapy to 4 cycles unless a significant response is clinically important, and in that case not treating with more than six cycles, is a reasonable strategy.

5.6.7 Maintenance therapy

A recent phase III study evaluated the use of maintenance chemotherapy in patients who completed their first line of therapy without disease progression. In a study of 663 patients who completed first line therapy with a non-pemetrexed containing platinum-based doublet without evidence of disease progression, subjects were randomized to receive maintenance treatment with pemetrexed plus best supportive care or to receive placebo plus best supportive care

Table 5.2 Select Phase 3 trials with single agent EGFR TKIs						
Trial	Treat-ment arms	TKI Treat-ment line	Patient cohort	Source	# pts	Result
BR21	Erlotinib vs placebo	2nd or 3rd line	NSCLC failed prior platinum	Ref. 13	N=731	6.7 m. vs 4.7 m. (p <.001)
INTEREST	Gefitinib vs do-cetaxel	2nd line	NSCLC	Ref. 48	N=1433	Non-inferiority
IPASS	Gefitinib vs carbo/tax	1st line	Asian never smokers or light former smokers*	Ref. 20	N=1217	PFS HR .741 (p<.0001)
IPASS Subset Analysis	Gefitinib vs carbo/tax	1st line	EGFR activating mutation subset	Ref. 20	261	PFS HR .48 (p<.0001)
Carbo/tax = carboplatin/taxol						

until disease progression. Patients who were randomized to maintenance pemetrexed had an improved overall survival of 13.4 months versus 10.6 months in the control arm (Ciuleanu *et al.*, 2008), and consequently, pemetrexed has been approved as maintenance therapy by the FDA. A concern identified in a study of this design is that not all patients assigned to the control arm went on to receive second-line therapy at all (only 18% of patients on the control arm went on to receive pemetrexed); therefore, it may not be the immediate use of pemetrexed that is beneficial to patients, but that they receive pemetrexed at any time after successful completion of their first line of therapy.

5.7 Poor performance status

Data is limited in patients with poor performance status, and their tolerance of combination chemotherapy is poor (Schiller *et al.*, 2002); therefore, alternate strategies should be employed when treating these patients with advanced disease.

Figure 5.1 Treatment algorithm

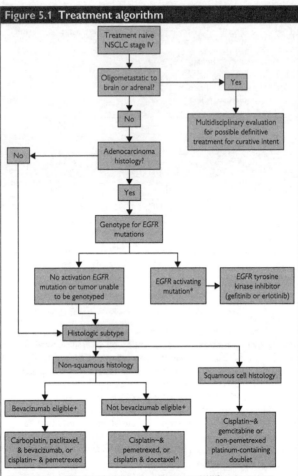

* Sensitizing mutations in EGFR include in-frame deletions in exon 19, missense exon 21 L858R mutations, or missense G719 mutations.

+Patients are considered ineligilbe to receive bevacizumab if they have squamous histology, are receiving full-dose anticoagulation, have unstable or untreated brain metastases, have a history of more than 1/2 tsp hemoptysis per episode in the previous 3 months, have had recent hemorrhage, have a history of coagulopathy or bleeding diasthesis, or have significant vascular disease.

^Cisplatin and pemetrexed has not been compared to cisplatin and docetaxel in treatment naive patients; however, in the second-line, single agent pemetrexed was found to be equivalent to docetaxel with less toxicity.

~Cisplatin appears to have a superior response rate to carboplatin, although it does not appear to improve overall survival.

Combination or single agent therapies are a reasonable treatment for patients with poor performance status (Lilenbaum et al., 2005; Hainsworth et al., 2007). For unselected patients, single agent docetaxel, vinorelbine, and gemcitabine have all been used with modest activity. Patients with EGFR-activating mutations who were not eligible for chemotherapy and were treated with EGFR tyrosine kinase inhibitors can have a 'Lazarus Response,' as amiably described by one reviewer, with a 66% response rate and 79% of patients had an improvement in performance status (Inoue et al., 2009); Langer, 2009). In a randomized study comparing erlotinib to carboplatin and paclitaxel in 103 unselected, treatment-naïve patients with ECOG performance status 2, the patients that received carboplatin and paclitaxel had an improved overall survival compared to erlotinib (9.7 mos vs 6.5 mos, HR for progression with erlotinib 1.73, P=.018) (Lilenbaum et al., 2008). Therefore, in patients with performance status 2, if they are EGFR wild-type or unable to be genotyped, and are appropriate for chemotherapy, chemotherapy may offer an improved survival over erlotinib. In patients that are EGFR mutant, however, erlotinib or gefitinib can offer a significant improvement in performance status.

Further reading

Asahina H., Yamazaki K., Kinoshita I., et al. (2006) A phase II trial of gefitinib as first-line therapy for advanced non-small cell lung cancer with epidermal growth factor receptor mutations. Br J Cancer **95**(8): 998–1004.

Billing P.S., Miller D.L., Allen M.S., Deschamps C., Trastek V.F., Pairolero P.C. (2001) Surgical treatment of primary lung cancer with synchronous brain metastases. J Thorac Cardiovasc Surg **122**(3): 548–53.

Ceppi P., Volante M., Saviozzi S., et al. (2006) Squamous cell carcinoma of the lung compared with other histotypes shows higher messenger RNA and protein levels for thymidylate synthase. Cancer **107**(7): 1589–96.

NSCLC Meta-Analyses Collaborative Group (2008) Chemotherapy in addition to supportive care improves survival in advanced non-small-cell lung cancer: a systematic review and meta-analysis of individual patient data from 16 randomized controlled trials. J Clin Oncol **26**(28): 4617–25.

Non-small Cell Lung Cancer Collaborative Group (1993) Chemotherapy in non-small cell lung cancer: a meta-analysis using updated data on individual patients from 52 randomised clinical trials. BMJ **11**(7010): 899–909.

Ciuleanu T.E., Brodowicz T., Belani C.P., et al. (2008) Maintenance pemetrexed plus best supportive care (BSC) versus placebo plus BSC: A phase III study. J Clin Oncol **26s**: abstr 8011.

Flannery T.W., Suntharalingam M., Regine W.F., *et al.* (2008) Long-term survival in patients with synchronous, solitary brain metastasis from non-small-cell lung cancer treated with radiosurgery. *Int J Radiat Oncol Biol Phys* **72**(1): 19–23.

Fossella F., Pereira J.R., von Pawel J., *et al.* (2003) Randomized, multinational, phase III study of docetaxel plus platinum combinations versus vinorelbine plus cisplatin for advanced non-small-cell lung cancer: the TAX 326 study group. *J Clin Oncol* **21**(16): 3016–24.

Fujino S., Enokibori T., Tezuka N., *et al.* (1996) A comparison of epidermal growth factor receptor levels and other prognostic parameters in non-small cell lung cancer. *Eur J Cancer* **32A**(12): 2070–4.

Gabrijel S., Grize L., Helfenstein E., *et al.* (2008) Receiving the diagnosis of lung cancer: patient recall of information and satisfaction with physician communication. *J Clin Oncol* ;**26**(2): 297–302.

Gatzemeier U., Pluzanska A., Szczesna A., *et al.* (2007) Phase III study of erlotinib in combination with cisplatin and gemcitabine in advanced non-small-cell lung cancer: the Tarceva Lung Cancer Investigation Trial. *J Clin Oncol* **25**(12): 1545–52.

Giaccone G., Herbst R.S., Manegold C., *et al.* (2004) Gefitinib in combination with gemcitabine and cisplatin in advanced non-small-cell lung cancer: a phase III trial—INTACT 1. *J Clin Oncol* **22**(5): 777–84.

Hainsworth J.D., Spigel D.R., Farley C., *et al.* (2007) Weekly docetaxel versus docetaxel/gemcitabine in the treatment of elderly or poor performance status patients with advanced nonsmall cell lung cancer: a randomized phase 3 trial of the Minnie Pearl Cancer Research Network. *Cancer* **110**(9): 2027–34.

Hanna N., Shepherd F.A., Fossella F.V., *et al.* (2004) Randomized phase III trial of pemetrexed versus docetaxel in patients with non-small-cell lung cancer previously treated with chemotherapy. *J Clin Oncol* **22**(9): 1589–97.

Herbst R.S., Giaccone G., Schiller J.H., *et al.* (2004) Gefitinib in combination with paclitaxel and carboplatin in advanced non-small-cell lung cancer: a phase III trial—INTACT 2. *J Clin Oncol* **22**(5): 785–94.

Herbst R.S., Prager D., Hermann R., *et al.* (2005) TRIBUTE: a phase III trial of erlotinib hydrochloride (OSI-774) combined with carboplatin and paclitaxel chemotherapy in advanced non-small-cell lung cancer. *J Clin Oncol* **23**(25): 5892–9.

Hu C., Chang E.L., Hassenbusch S.J., 3rd, *et al.* (2006) Nonsmall cell lung cancer presenting with synchronous solitary brain metastasis. *Cancer* **106**(9): 1998–2004.

Inoue A., Kobayashi K., Usui K., *et al.* (2009) First-line gefitinib for patients with advanced non-small-cell lung cancer harboring epidermal growth factor receptor mutations without indication for chemotherapy. *J Clin Oncol* **27**(9): 1394–1400.

Inoue A., Suzuki T., Fukuhara T., *et al.* (2006) Prospective phase II study of gefitinib for chemotherapy-naive patients with advanced non-small-cell lung cancer with epidermal growth factor receptor gene mutations. *J Clin Oncol* **24**(21): 3340–6.

Jemal A., Siegel R., Ward E., Hao Y., Xu J., Thun M.J. (2009) Cancer statistics, 2009. *CA Cancer J Clin* **59**(4): 225–49.

Johnson D.H., Fehrenbacher L., Novotny W.F., *et al.* (2004) Randomized phase II trial comparing bevacizumab plus carboplatin and paclitaxel with carboplatin and paclitaxel alone in previously untreated locally advanced or metastatic non-small-cell lung cancer. *J Clin Oncol* **22**(11): 2184–91.

Kim E.S., Hirsh V., Mok T., *et al.* (2008) Gefitinib versus docetaxel in previously treated non-small-cell lung cancer (INTEREST): a randomised phase III trial. *Lancet* **372**(9652): 1809–18.

Langer C.J. (2009) The 'lazarus response' in treatment-naive, poor performance status patients with non-small-cell lung cancer and epidermal growth factor receptor mutation. *J Clin Oncol* **27**(9): 1350–4.

Lilenbaum R., Axelrod R., Thomas S., *et al.* (2008) Randomized phase II trial of erlotinib or standard chemotherapy in patients with advanced non-small-cell lung cancer and a performance status of 2. *J Clin Oncol* **26**(6): 863–9.

Lilenbaum R.C., Herndon J.E., 2nd, List M.A., *et al.* (2005) Single-agent versus combination chemotherapy in advanced non-small-cell lung cancer: the cancer and leukemia group B (study 9730). *J Clin Oncol* **23**(1): 190–6.

Lynch T., Bell D.W., Sordella R., *et al.* (2004) Activating mutations in the epidermal growth factor receptor underlying responsiveness of non-small-cell lung cancer to gefitinib. *N Engl J Med* **350**(21): 2129–39.

Mattern J., Koomagi R., Volm M. (1996) Association of vascular endothelial growth factor expression with intratumoral microvessel density and tumour cell proliferation in human epidermoid lung carcinoma. *Br J Cancer* **73**(7): 931–4.

Mok T.S., Wu Y.L., Thongprasert S., *et al.* (2009) Gefitinib or Carboplatin-Paclitaxel in Pulmonary Adenocarcinoma. *N Engl J Med*.

Paez J.G., Janne P.A., Lee J.C., *et al.* (2004) EGFR mutations in lung cancer: correlation with clinical response to gefitinib therapy. *Science* **304**(5676): 1497–1500.

Pao W., Miller V., Zakowski M., *et al.* (2004) EGF receptor gene mutations are common in lung cancers from 'never smokers' and are associated with sensitivity of tumors to gefitinib and erlotinib. *Proc Natl Acad Sci USA* **101**(36): 13306–11.

Patel J.D., Bonomi P., Socinski M.A., *et al.* (2009) Treatment rationale and study design for the pointbreak study: a randomized, open-label phase III study of pemetrexed/carboplatin/bevacizumab followed by maintenance pemetrexed/bevacizumab versus paclitaxel/carboplatin/bevacizumab followed by maintenance bevacizumab in patients with stage IIIB or IV nonsquamous non-small-cell lung cancer. *Clin Lung Cancer* **10**(4): 252–6.

Pirker R., Pereira J.R., Szczesna A., *et al.* (2009) Cetuximab plus chemotherapy in patients with advanced non-small-cell lung cancer (FLEX): an open-label randomised phase III trial. *Lancet* **373**(9674): 1525–31.

Salomon D.S., Brandt R., Ciardiello F., Normanno N. (1995) Epidermal growth factor-related peptides and their receptors in human malignancies. *Crit Rev Oncol Hematol* **19**(3): 183–232.

Sandler A., Gray R., Perry M.C., *et al.* (2006) Paclitaxel-carboplatin alone or with bevacizumab for non-small-cell lung cancer. *N Engl J Med* **355**(24): 2542–50.

Scagliotti G., Hanna N., Fossella F., *et al.* (2009)The differential efficacy of pemetrexed according to NSCLC histology: a review of two Phase III studies. *Oncologist* **14**(3): 253–63.

Scagliotti G.V., Parikh P., von Pawel J., *et al.* (2008) Phase III study comparing cisplatin plus gemcitabine with cisplatin plus pemetrexed in chemotherapy-naive patients with advanced-stage non-small-cell lung cancer. *J Clin Oncol* **26**(21): 3543–51.

Schiller J.H., Harrington D., Belani C.P., *et al.* (2002) Comparison of four chemotherapy regimens for advanced non-small-cell lung cancer *N Engl J Med* **346**(2): 92–8.

Sequist L.V., Martins R.G., Spigel D., *et al.* (2008) First-line gefitinib in patients with advanced non-small-cell lung cancer harboring somatic EGFR mutations. *J Clin Oncol* **26**(15): 2442–49.

Shepherd F.A., Rodrigues Pereira J., Ciuleanu T., *et al.* (2005) Erlotinib in previously treated non-small-cell lung cancer. *N Engl J Med* **353**(2): 123–32.

Smith I.E., O'Brien M.E., Talbot D.C., *et al.* (2001) Duration of chemotherapy in advanced non-small-cell lung cancer: a randomized trial of three versus six courses of mitomycin, vinblastine, and cisplatin. *J Clin Oncol* **19**(5): 1336–43.

Socinski M.A., Langer C.J., Huang J.E., *et al.* (2009) Safety of bevacizumab in patients with non-small-cell lung cancer and brain metastases. *J Clin Oncol* **27**(31): 5255–61.

Socinski M.A., Schell M.J., Peterman A., *et al.* (2002) Phase III trial comparing a defined duration of therapy versus continuous therapy followed by second-line therapy in advanced-stage IIIB/IV non-small-cell lung cancer. *J Clin Oncol* **20**(5): 1335–43.

Spiro S.G., Rudd R.M., Souhami R.L., *et al.* (2004) Chemotherapy versus supportive care in advanced non-small cell lung cancer: improved survival without detriment to quality of life. *Thorax* **59**(10): 828–38.

Sugimura H., Nichols F.C., Yang P., *et al.* (2007) Survival after recurrent non small-cell lung cancer after complete pulmonary resection. *Ann Thorac Surg* **83**(2): 409–17; discussion 417–18.

Tanvetyanon T., Robinson L.A., Schell M.J., *et al.* (2008) Outcomes of adrenalectomy for isolated synchronous versus metachronous adrenal metastases in non-small-cell lung cancer: a systematic review and pooled analysis. *J Clin Oncol* **26**(7): 1142–7.

Thatcher N., Chang A., Parikh P., *et al.* (2005) Gefitinib plus best supportive care in previously treated patients with refractory advanced non-small-cell lung cancer: results from a randomised, placebo-controlled, multicentre study (Iressa Survival Evaluation in Lung Cancer). *Lancet* **366**(9496): 1527–37.

Twomey P., Montgomery C., Clark O. (1982) Successful treatment of adrenal metastases from large-cell carcinoma of the lung. *JAMA* **248**(5): 581–3.

von Plessen C., Bergman B., Andresen O., *et al.* (2006) Palliative chemotherapy beyond three courses conveys no survival or consistent quality-of-life benefits in advanced non-small-cell lung cancer. *Br J Cancer* **95**(8): 966–73.

Chapter 6

Systemic therapy for recurrent NSCLC, efficacy, and toxicity

Paul Wheatley-Price and Frances A. Shepherd

Key points

- Patients with advanced non-small-cell lung cancer are destined to progress at some point following first-line therapy
- There are now multiple options for clinicians in the treatment of recurrent disease, using cytotoxic or biological therapies
- Docetaxel, pemetrexed, erlotinib and gefitinib all have phase III trial evidence supporting their use, and multiple other agents or combinations are being studied
- Identifiable patient and tumour characteristics will increasingly help to guide the selection of therapy in these patients.

6.1 Introduction

Platinum-based chemotherapy is the standard of care for fit patients with advanced non-small-cell lung cancer (NSCLC). However, almost all patients subsequently relapse and die of their disease, with few patients surviving beyond 2 years. Until recently, few patients received second-line therapy. Reasons for this included the reduced performance status of patients with progressive disease, but also the lack of efficacious second-line treatments. In fact, second-line chemotherapy has only become an accepted standard of care in the past decade.

In this chapter the role of systemic therapy for patients with progressive NSCLC after failure of first-line treatment is reviewed. The focus is on drugs for which phase III randomized trials support their use. A selection of promising drugs and targets that are being investigated are also discussed.

6.2 Chemotherapy

Two cytotoxic agents, docetaxel and pemetrexed, are approved for recurrent NSCLC after prior platinum-based therapy. Other single agents have been tested in phase III trials but have not demonstrated a sufficiently improved efficacy or toxicity profile to be adopted widely (Table 6.1). Only one phase III study (terminated early), and a number of randomized phase II studies, have tested single agent *versus* doublet therapies. Currently there is insufficient evidence to support doublet therapy, which generally is associated with increased toxicity without an accompanying improvement in response or survival. In a review of 19 phase III second-line chemotherapy trials in NSCLC published by Hotta et al., the overall response rate was 6.8% with a median survival of 6.6 months.

6.2.1 Docetaxel

In 2000, Shepherd *et al.* published the first clinical trial that demonstrated a survival benefit from second-line therapy. TAX317 was an international study that randomized patients, previously treated with platinum-based chemotherapy, to receive 3-weekly docetaxel 100 mg/m^2 (n = 49), and following a protocol amendment, docetaxel 75 mg/m^2 (n = 55), or best supportive care (BSC) (n = 100). Treatment continued until disease progression. The response rate in the combined docetaxel arms was 5.8% with no responding patient having progressed while on platinum chemotherapy; all responders had a good performance status (PS) (Eastern Cooperative Oncology Group [ECOG] 0–1). Docetaxel treatment was associated with longer survival than BSC (7.0 *versus* 4.6 months, p = 0.047). When comparing the two docetaxel dose groups with BSC individually, only those treated at 75 mg/m^2 had a significant survival advantage over supportive care (7.5 *versus* 4.6 months, p = 0.01). At 75 mg/m^2, neutropenia was seen in 67.3% of patients, but the incidence of febrile neutropenia was only 1.8%, compared to 22.4% at the 100mg/m^2 dose. No non-hematological toxicities were observed at significantly increased levels in the docetaxel arm compared to BSC.

Supporting data for the use of docetaxel 75 mg/m^2 came from the TAX 320 study reported by Fossella et al., in which patients were randomized to receive docetaxel 100 mg/m^2 *versus* docetaxel 75 mg/m^2 *versus* a control arm of vinorelbine or ifosfamide. While overall survival was not significantly different among the groups, docetaxel was associated with significantly higher response rates at both dose levels. Furthermore, patients receiving docetaxel 75 mg/m^2 had the greatest 1-year survival rate, and treatment was well tolerated at this lower dose.

Table 6.1 Response and survival in phase III chemotherapy trials for recurrent NSCLC

Study	Treatment	ORR (%)	Median PFS (months)	Median OS (months)	HR (95% CI) for OS
TAX317	Docetaxel 100mg/m^2	6.3		5.9	Not reported
	Docetaxel 75mg/m^2	5.5		7.5	
	Best supportive care	–		4.6	
TAX320	Docetaxel 100mg/m^2	10.8	1.9	5.5	Not reported
	Docetaxel 75mg/m^2	6.7	2.0	5.7	
	Vinorelbine/ ifosfamide	0.8	1.8	5.6	
Hanna et al.	Docetaxel 75mg/m^2	8.8	2.9	7.9	0.99 (0.8 – 1.2) p=0.23
	Pemetrexed 500mg/m^2	9.1	2.9	8.3	
Cullen et al.	Pemetrexed 500mg/m^2	7.1	2.6	6.7	1.01 (0.84 – 1.23)
	Pemetrexed 900mg/m^2	4.3	2.8	6.9	
Ramlau et al.	Docetaxel 75mg/m^2	4	3.0	7.2	1.23 (1.06 – 1.44) p=0.06
	Oral topotecan 2.3mg/m^2 days 1–5	5	2.5	6.5	
Krzakowski et al.	Docetaxel 75mg/m^2	5.5	2.3	7.2	0.97 (0.81 – 1.18)
	Vinflunine 320mg/m^2	4.4	2.3	6.7	
STELLAR-2	Docetaxel 75mg/m^2	12	2.6*	6.9	1.09 (0.94 – 1.27) p=0.26
	Paclitaxel poliglumex 210mg/m^2 in PS1 175mg/m^2 in PS2	8	2.0*	6.9	

PS1 = performance status 1; PS2 = performance status 2

As a result of these studies, docetaxel 75 mg/m^2 every 3 weeks became the treatment of choice for recurrent NSCLC, and continues to represent a standard against which other regimens are measured.

Several studies have investigated the weekly administration of docetaxel with doses ranging from 33.3 mg/m^2 to 40 mg/m^2. In an individual patient data meta-analysis, including five of these randomized trials, median survival was similar regardless of schedule, but significantly lower rates of neutropenia and febrile neutropenia were seen with the weekly schedules. Weekly docetaxel, therefore, is a reasonable alternative to 3-weekly administration, although this should be balanced against the convenience of a 3-weekly schedule.

6.2.2 **Pemetrexed**

Pemetrexed is a multitargeted antifolate cytotoxic agent. In combination with cisplatin it is licensed in the first-line treatment of NSCLC in non-squamous histologies. Folate and vitamin B$_{12}$ supplementation is required with pemetrexed, to reduce the incidence of both hematological and non-hematological toxicities. In a 571 patient phase III trial with a non-inferiority design, reported by Hanna et al., pemetrexed 500mg/m^2 was compared to docetaxel 75 mg/m^2. Patients, of ECOG PS 0-2 and previously treated with *only one regimen* of chemotherapy, were treated until progression or unacceptable toxicity. Response rates were similar between the arms (pemetrexed 9.1%, docetaxel 8.8%). The primary outcome measure, overall survival, was not significantly different between treatments (hazard ratio [HR] 0.99, 95% confidence interval [CI] 0.82–1.20, non-inferiority p = 0.23). Prior treatment with first-line paclitaxel did not noticeably affect outcomes from second-line docetaxel, a finding also seen in TAX320.

Although the efficacy of the two drugs was similar, those receiving docetaxel had significantly higher rates of neutropenia, febrile neutropenia, requirement for granulocyte colony stimulating factor and hospitalization.

In an attempt to improve the efficacy of pemetrexed, a phase III trial randomized patients to either 500 mg/m^2 (n = 295) or 900 mg/m^2 (n = 293). At the higher dose there was no significant improvement in response rate, progression free survival (PFS) or overall survival (HR 1.01, 95%CI 0.84–1.23, p = 0.89). Patients treated with 900 mg/m^2 experienced higher rates of neutropenia, thrombocytopenia and fatigue. Therefore, pemetrexed 500 mg/m^2 remains the recommended dose in this setting.

Recently, it has been demonstrated that there is differential benefit to pemetrexed according to histological subtype. Both the first-line study that compared cisplatin-pemetrexed with cisplatin-gemcitabine, and the second-line study, suggested that patients with non-squamous cancers had longer survival if treated with pemetrexed, whereas those with squamous cell carcinoma survived longer if treated with the alternate agents. The biological rationale for this difference may be due to differential expression of thymidylate synthase (TS), a prime target of pemetrexed, in squamous and non-squamous carcinomas.

Scagliotti *et al.* reported that, in the second-line trial, there was a significant treatment-histology interaction (interaction p = 0.001). Patients with non-squamous carcinoma had significantly longer survival if treated with pemetrexed (HR 0.78, 95%CI 0.61–1.00, p = 0.047), whereas those with squamous carcinoma had significantly *shorter* survival if treated with pemetrexed (HR 1.56, 95%CI 1.08–2.26; p = 0.018). The efficacy of docetaxel, however, did not alter according to histological type. The treatment-by-histology analyses of the second-line trial were performed retrospectively, but similar significant interaction also has been reported in trials comparing pemetrexed and cisplatin to gemcitabine and cisplatin in the first-line setting, and maintenance pemetrexed compared to placebo in patients responding to first-line doublet chemotherapy. As a result of these trials and subsequent analyses, pemetrexed is considered an alternative standard of care in the treatment of recurrent NSCLC of non-squamous histology.

6.2.3 **Other chemotherapeutic agents**
While docetaxel and pemetrexed are the only *cytotoxic* agents approved in recurrent NSCLC, other agents have been tested in second-line trials.

Ifosfamide and vinorelbine were compared to docetaxel in the TAX320 study, as previously discussed.

In an 829 patient phase III trial comparing oral topotecan to docetaxel 75 mg/m^2, response rates were similar between groups. However overall survival was shorter in the topotecan arm (HR 1.16, 95%CI 1.00–1.35, p = 0.057); therefore neither the oral nor the intravenous formulation of topotecan has been adopted into widespread usage.

Another phase III trial randomized patients with recurrent NSCLC to vinflunine 320 mg/m^2 (n = 274) or docetaxel 75 mg/m^2 (n=277). This was a non-inferiority study, with PFS as the primary endpoint. There were no significant differences between treatments with respect to response, PFS or overall survival. Toxicities were similar, although slightly more grade 3 or 4 anemia, leucopenia, thrombocytopenia, and fatigue were seen in patients treated with vinflunine.

The STELLAR-2 study randomized 849 patients to receive docetaxel 75 mg/m^2 or paclitaxel poliglumex, a novel paclitaxel formulation designed to reduce toxicity. The trial was designed to demonstrate the superiority of paclitaxel poliglumex; however, median overall survival was 6.9 months in both arms. Patients treated with paclitaxel poliglumex experienced significantly lower rates of neutropenia, febrile neutropenia, alopecia, fatigue, and mucositis. While not yet routinely used or widely available, the favourable toxicity profile makes paclitaxel poliglumex a potentially attractive alternative to docetaxel.

6.3 **Biological therapy**

Erlotinib and gefitinib are oral small molecule tyrosine kinase inhibitors (TKIs) of the epidermal growth factor receptor (EGFR) pathway. They have been studied in combination with chemotherapy in several large phase III trials in the first-line setting, but none demonstrated improved efficacy outcomes compared to chemotherapy alone. However both of these drugs have demonstrated efficacy in recurrent NSCLC (Table 6.2), and their toxicity profiles compare favourably with cytoptoxic therapy (Table 6.3).

Table 6.2 Response and survival from phase III trials of epidermal growth factor tyrosine kinase inhibitors in recurrent NSCLC

Study	Treatment	ORR (%)	Median PFS (months)	Median OS (months)	HR (95% CI) for OS
BR.21	Erlotinib	8.9	2.2	6.7	0.70 (0.58 – 0.85) p<0.001
	Best supportive care	<1	1.8	4.7	
ISEL	Gefitinib	8	3.0*	5.6	0.89 (0.77 – 1.02) p=0.09
	Best supportive care	1	2.6*	5.1	
INTEREST	Gefitinib	9.1	2.2	7.6	1.02 (0.91 – 1.15)
	Docetaxel	7.6	2.7	8.0	
BETA	Erlotinib/ placebo	6.2	1.7	9.2	0.97 p=0.76
	Erlotinib/ bevacizumab	12.6	3.4	9.3	
ZEST	Vandetanib	12	2.6	6.9	1.01 (0.89 – 1.16) p=0.83
	Erlotinib	12	2.1	7.8	
ZEAL	Pemetrexed/ vandetanib	19.1	4.1	10.5	0.86 (0.65 – 1.13) p=0.22
	Pemetrexed/ placebo	7.9	2.7	9.2	
ZODIAC	Docetaxel/ vandetanib	17	4.0	10.6	0.91 (0.78 – 1.07) p=0.20
	Docetaxel/ placebo	10	3.2	10.0	

Table 6.3 A comparison of common serious toxicities (grade 3-4) for the currently approved agents

Toxicity	Docetaxel	Pemetrexed	Erlotinib	Gefitinib
Neutropenia	40.2–67.3%	5.3%	–	2.2%
Febrile neutropenia	1.8–12.7%	1.9%	–	1.2%
Vomiting	1–3.6%	1.5%	3%	0.5–1%
Fatigue	5.4–18.2%	5.3%	19%	3–4.4%
Neuropathy	1–2.4%	0.0%	–	0.1%
Rash	0.6–0.7%	0.8%	9%	2–2.1%
Diarrhoea	1.8–3.1%	0.4%	6%	2.5–3%

[1] From TAX 317, TAX 320, Hanna et al. and INTEREST, refers to 75mg/m^2 3-weekly;
[2] From Hanna et al;. [3] From BR.21; [4] From ISEL and INTEREST

6.3.1 **Erlotinib**

The BR.21 study randomized 731 patients who were not eligible for further chemotherapy, to either erlotinib (n = 488) or placebo (n = 243). Approximately half the patients were treated in the second-line and half in the third-line setting. The response rate was 8.9% in the erlotinib arm, and survival was significantly prolonged by erlotinib (HR 0.70, 95%CI 0.58-0.85, p<0.001). Asian origin, adenocarcinoma, female sex and a history of never smoking were associated with higher response rates, but the only clinical factor associated with a differential survival benefit was smoking history. Treatment with erlotinib was associated with improved quality-of-life.

In some countries, erlotinib approval is restricted to the population of patients defined by the BR.21 trial, and so it is administered as third-line treatment after two lines of chemotherapy or as second-line treatment in patients not eligible for further chemotherapy. However, it is also used as the treatment of choice *before* second-line chemotherapy by many physicians, although there are no data available yet to support its use in this setting. Ongoing phase III trials, including TITAN and the North American VITAL study are comparing erlotinib with either docetaxel or pemetrexed. Results of these trials are awaited.

In the future patients may be selected for treatment with EGFR TKIs on the basis of their tumour molecular status in addition to clinical factors. Zhu et al. published an analysis of *KRAS* and *EGFR* status from BR.21. Patients with wild-type *KRAS* had a significant survival benefit when treated with erlotinib (HR 0.69, p=0.03), whereas no benefit was seen in *KRAS* mutant patients. Patients with either FISH-positive *EGFR* status or an *EGFR* mutation had higher response rates to erlotinib than *EGFR* FISH-negative or *EGFR* wild-type patients. A significant survival benefit from erlotinib was seen in

EGFR FISH-positive patients (HR 0.43, p = 0.004) but not FISH-negative patients. Patients with EGFR wild-type and mutant tumours both appeared to benefit from erlotinib, with no *significant* interaction demonstrated for mutation status.

6.3.2 **Gefitinib**

The ISEL study, similar in design to BR.21, compared gefitinib to BSC in patients who were either refractory to, or intolerant of chemotherapy. However in contrast to BR.21, gefitinib did not show an overall survival benefit, although significantly longer survival was seen amongst Asians and never-smokers. Thus, gefitinib was not approved in Europe or North America, although it is used widely in Asian countries. Reasons why ISEL was negative are unclear, but possibly relate to the best response to prior therapy (38% in BR.21, 18% in ISEL) indicating more refractory patients in ISEL.

EGFR analyses for ISEL were published by Hirsch *et al.* High *EGFR* copy number was associated with improved survival from gefitinib compared to placebo (HR 0.61, p = 0.07). While *EGFR* mutations were associated with a higher response rate, there were too few events to analyse the effect on survival.

Gefitinib has been compared to second-line *chemotherapy* in several randomized phase II and III trials. INTEREST, the largest of these, was an international trial that randomized patients, pre-treated with platinum-based chemotherapy, to receive docetaxel 75 mg/m^2 every 3 weeks (n = 733) or gefitinib 250 mg daily (n = 733). The study achieved its primary endpoint in demonstrating *non-inferiority* of overall survival for gefitinib compared to docetaxel (HR 1.02, 95%CI 0.90–1.15). Response rates were similar (9.1% *versus* 7.6%, p = 0.33). Gefitinib was better tolerated than docetaxel, with significantly lower rates of serious adverse events (4% *versus* 18%), particularly lower rates of neutropenia, febrile neutropenia, stomatitis, neurotoxicity and myalgia. As expected diarrhea and skin rash were more common in patients receiving gefitinib. Improvements in quality of life (25% *versus* 15%, p<0.0001) and in lung cancer symptoms (20% *versus* 17%, p = 0.13) were more common in the gefitinib arm.

In INTEREST there were no significant differences in the survival results in pre-planned subgroup analyses based on performance status, histology, smoking history, sex, age and ethnicity. Furthermore, unlike the results seen in the placebo-controlled studies, EGFR status (gene copy number, protein expression or mutation status) and *KRAS* mutation status did not influence the survival results.

In addition to INTEREST, three smaller studies also have investigated gefitinib *versus* docetaxel in recurrent disease (SIGN, V15–32 and ISTANA). A meta-analysis of these trials, with 2,224 patients, confirmed non-inferiority of gefitinib in this setting (HR for survival

1.03, 95% CI 9.93–1.13). On the basis of these results, gefitinib is a valid alternative to docetaxel in the treatment of recurrent NSCLC.

6.4 **Future directions**

Bevacizumab, a monoclonal antibody that targets vascular endothelial growth factor (VEGF), has phase III trial evidence demonstrating efficacy in the first-line treatment of NSCLC. In a *second-line* randomized phase II trial that compared bevacizumab plus docetaxel or pemetrexed *versus* bevacizumab plus erlotinib *versus* docetaxel or pemetrexed plus placebo, a trend towards improved survival was reported in the bevacizumab-containing cohorts, with lower toxicity observed in the bevacizumab/erlotinib arm. However, the confirmatory phase III BeTa lung trial, that randomized previously treated NSCLC patients to erlotinib plus bevacizumab *versus* erlotinib alone, demonstrated no survival benefit from the addition of bevacizumab (HR 0.97, p = 0.76), although overall response rates were higher (12.6% *versus* 6.2%, p=0.006) and PFS was longer (HR 0.62, p<0.001).

Another angiogenesis inhibitor, the fusion protein aflibercept (VEGF-trap), is being evaluated in a phase III trial of docetaxel +/- aflibercept in patients with non-squamous tumours. A similar phase III trial of docetaxel +/-the vascular disrupting agent ASA-404 is ongoing. Cediranib, sorafenib, pazopanib and BIBF-1120 are also being tested in recurrent NSCLC.

Vandetanib is a small molecule inhibitor of both EGFR and VEGF that has been studied in a series of randomized trials in recurrent NSCLC. In a head-to-head trial *versus* erlotinib (ZEST) there was no difference in PFS or overall survival, but more patients receiving vandetanib experienced ≥grade 3 toxicities. Further trials have compared the combination of vandetanib and docetaxel (ZODIAC) or pemetrexed (ZEAL) *versus* chemotherapy alone. Longer PFS was seen in patients treated with vandetanib/docetaxel compared to docetaxel monotherapy, but there was no significant difference in overall survival. No significant difference in either PFS or OS was observed in ZEAL.

A number of other agents are being investigated in recurrent disease. Molecules that target EGFR and other receptors of the EGFR family include EKB-569, CL-387785, HKI-272, BIBW-2992, PKI-166, CI-1033 and PF-00299804. In particular those that are irreversible inhibitors of EGFR appear promising, with the potential to overcome resistance to erlotinib or gefitinib. Two of these agents, BIBW-2992 and PF-00299804 are being compared to placebo in randomized trials in the third-line or fourth-line setting. The EGFR monoclonal antibody cetuximab also is under investigation with both docetaxel and pemetrexed.

Alternative molecular targets of therapeutic interest include the mammalian target of rapamycin (mTOR), the proteosome, or insulin growth factor receptor (IGFR). The mTOR inhibitor RAD-001 (everolimus) is being studied in combination with pemetrexed, docetaxel and the two EGFR TKIs, erlotinib and gefitinib in the second- and third-line settings. The proteosome inhibitor bortezomib was evaluated in a randomized trial that compared the combination of bortezomib and docetaxel to bortezomib alone. Single agent bortezomib was inferior to the combination, and the combination arm did not appear to produce results that were superior to those achieved with single-agent docetaxel. IGF1-R inhibitors may be of particular interest as they appear to be active against squamous cell cancers, and randomized trials evaluating several agents in this class are ongoing in the first-line and second-line settings. The MET inhibitor PF-02341066 may be particularly active against the small population of patients with the EML4/ALK fusion gene, and finally, the MEK inhibitor AZD6224 also is under evaluation with docetaxel in a randomized phase II trial.

6.5 **Conclusions**

On the basis of current evidence, docetaxel, pemetrexed and gefitinib have phase III trial evidence to support their use in the second-line setting after first-line platinum-based chemotherapy. In addition both erlotinib and gefitinib have phase III trial evidence supporting their use in the second- or third-line setting, when chemotherapy is no longer indicated.

The choice of which drug to select should be based on patient and tumour characteristics. Patients with squamous cell carcinoma should not receive pemetrexed, but for other cell types docetaxel or pemetrexed may be considered. Gefitinib and erlotinib, while showing improved response rates in adenocarcinoma, also demonstrate efficacy in patients with squamous cell histology based on subgroup analyses.

At the molecular level, BR.21 and ISEL both showed that patients whose tumours had *EGFR* activating mutations and those with high *EGFR* copy number had higher response rates and a greater survival advantage compared to placebo. However, when these markers were evaluated in the INTEREST trial, they did not predict for a differential benefit for either EGFR TKI therapy or docetaxel chemotherapy. In all studies, biomarker analyses were performed retrospectively, and adequate samples for testing were available in only 20–30% of trial patients. Furthermore, even for the subset of patients with tissue available, samples were not collected at the time of treatment, and collection may have antedated the initiation of therapy by months and even years. The North American intergroup MARVEL trial is a biomarker validation study that is designed to determine *prospectively* whether *EGFR* copy number is a valid test to select patients for EGFR TKI therapy or chemotherapy in the second-line setting. However, emerging data from the I-PASS study in the first-line setting suggest that the EGFR TKI gefitinib may be a *preferred* treatment in patients with *EGFR* gene mutations, and so chemotherapy may become the only option for second-line therapy in these patients.

Another factor that clinicians should consider is performance status. Given the favorable toxicity profile of pemetrexed and the EGFR TKIs when compared to docetaxel, these options may be preferable in the more frail population.

Many clinicians may still elect to give a cytotoxic agent (docetaxel or pemetrexed) in the second-line setting *before* an EGFR TKI, sensing that patients may still be fit enough for the less toxic EGFR TKI as third-line therapy, thereby allowing their patients the maximum opportunity for three lines of treatment. However in INTERST, similar proportions of patients in each arm received third-line treatment.

Recent studies suggest that maintenance therapy with either single-agent chemotherapy or erlotinib after platinum-based treatment results in prolongation of PFS and in some cases survival. In the maintenance study of erlotinib (SATURN), the benefit in terms of prolongation of PFS was most marked in patients with *EGFR* sensitizing mutations. However, although the interaction was significant (interaction p-value<0.001), patients with both mutated *EGFR* (HR = 0.10, p<0.0001) and wild-type *EFGR* (HR = 0.78, p = 0.0185) derived significant survival benefit, indicating quantitative rather than qualitative interaction. Interestingly, no significant interaction was seen when overall survival was considered. With respect to maintenance pemetrexed, the overall survival benefit from maintenance therapy was seen *only* in patients with tumours of non-squamous histology where a clinically meaningful prolongation of median survival of 5 months was seen (median survival 15.5 *versus* 10.3 months, HR 0.70, p = 0.002). If maintenance (or early introduction of second-line therapy) becomes a new standard of care, fewer options will be available to patients who relapse after their first-line 'package' of therapy. In effect, these patients will be receiving third-line treatment at the time of progression after first-line induction followed by maintenance therapy, and new strategies may have to be explored.

It is interesting to reflect upon the unprecedented change that has taken place over the space of only 10 years in the treatment of advanced NSCLC. There are now approved agents that have the potential to prolong survival and improve symptoms and quality of life as first-, second- and even third-line therapy for this malignancy. This means that new agents for NSCLC must be introduced in the *fourth-line setting*, a concept that would have be unthinkable in the 1990s! Agents that are being evaluated as fourth-line treatment in randomized placebo controlled trials include the irreversible EGFR inhibitors PF-00299804 and BIBW-2992 and, the dual EGFR and VEGF inhibitor vandetanib. Studies of the latter two agents have completed accrual, but follow-up is still ongoing and results are not yet available.

In summary, there are now a number of alternatives for patients with recurrent disease after first-line systemic therapy. The development of new targets and agents is likely to mean that increasing numbers of patients will be able to benefit from second-, third- and perhaps even fourth-line treatments in the future.

Further reading

Di Maio M., Perrone F., Chiodini P., et al. (2007) Individual patient data meta-analysis of docetaxel administered once every 3 weeks compared with once every week second-line treatment of advanced non-small-cell lung cancer. J Clin Oncol **25**: 1377–82.

Fossella F., DeVore R., Kerr R.N., et al. (2000) Randomized phase III trial of docetaxel versus vinorelbine or ifosfamide in patients with advanced non-small cell lung cancer previously treated with platinum-containing chemotherapy regimens. J Clin Oncol **18**: 2354–62.

Hanna N., Shepherd F.A., Fossella F.V., et al. (2004) Randomized phase III trial of pemetrexed versus docetaxel in patients with non-small-cell lung cancer previously treated with chemotherapy. J Clin Oncol **22**: 1589–97.

Hotta K., Fujiwara Y., Kiura K., et al. (2007) Relationship between response and survival in more than 50,000 patients with advanced non-small cell lung cancer treated with systemic chemotherapy in 143 phase III trials. J Thorac Oncol **2**: 402–7.

Kim E., Hirsh V., Mok T., et al. (2008) Gefitinib versus docetaxel in previously treated non-small-cell lung cancer (INTEREST): a randomised phase III trial. Lancet **372**: 1809–18.

Scagliotti G., Hanna N., Fossella F., et al. (2009) The differential efficacy of pemetrexed according to NSCLC histology: A review of two phase III studies. The Oncologist **14**: 253–63.

Shepherd F.A., Dancey J., Ramlau R., et al. (2000) Prospective randomized trial of docetaxel versus best supportive care in patients with non-small-cell lung cancer previously treated with platinum-based chemotherapy. J Clin Oncol **18**: 2095–103.

Shepherd F.A., Rodrigues Pereira J., Ciuleanu T., et al. (2005) Erlotinib in previously treated non-small-cell lung cancer. N Engl J Med **353**: 123–32.

Thatcher N., Chang A., Parikh P., et al. (2005) Gefitinib plus best supportive care in previously treated patients with refractory advanced non-small-cell lung cancer: results from a randomised, placebo-controlled, multicentre study (Iressa Survival Evaluation in Lung Cancer). Lancet **366**: 1527–37.

Wheatley-Price P. and Shepherd F.A. (2008) Epidermal growth factor receptor inhibitors in the treatment of lung cancer: reality and hopes. Curr Opin Oncol **20**: 162–75.

Wheatley-Price P. and Shepherd F.A. (2008) Targeting angiogenesis in the treatment of lung cancer. J Thorac Oncol **3**: 1173–84.

Chapter 7

Palliative care in NSCLC

Paul Baas and Wilma Uyterlinde

> **Key points**
> - The primary objective in patients with lung cancer is to improve Quality of Life
> - The treatment of cachexia in patients with lung cancer is limited and has not proven to improve survival
> - In the case of dyspnea, cough or hemoptysis, endobronchial examination should be performed besides symptom management
> - Radiation therapy can be used as simple and good palliation in symptomatic patients
> - Pleural effusions often occur during the course of the disease and should be managed immediately.

7.1 Introduction

Lung cancer patients may develop a variety of signs and symptoms during the course of the disease. Many of these symptoms result in a loss of quality of life and early implementation of palliative treatment is therefore of utmost importance. Some of these symptoms are directly related to the lung malignancy (e.g. hemoptysis, dyspnea, cough, pain, superior vena cava syndrome) or are related to systemic effects of the cancer (fatigue, anorexia, weakness, depression). The most frequent occurring symptoms are presented in this chapter and guidelines for treatment are given.

7.2 Pain

Patients with an advanced stage of lung cancer often experience moderate to severe pain. Pain can develop as a result of:
- Direct involvement or compression of structures that contain sensory nerves. This occurs most often due to direct growth into the parietal pleura or chest wall by the primary tumour
- Distant metastases (e.g. bone metastases, spinal cord compression, liver metastases)

• As a result of the treatment (esophagitis after radiation therapy or mucositis as a result of chemotherapy).

The assessment includes determination of the exact location and extent of the pain and the potential cause of the pain. The intensity of the pain can be evaluated using a pain scale. The primary goal of pain treatment is to treat the underlying cause and if this is not possible to increase the pain threshold.

7.2.1 **Localized pain**

In a case where the pain is localized the treatment options include radiation, intercostal nerve blocking, and cordotomy combined with oral or trans-cutaneous pain medication. Radiation is generally administered in limited number of fractions with a relatively high dose depending of the location, involved field and previous radiation treatment (e.g. 1 x 10Gy to 5 x 4Gy) In some cases the application of a local morphine gel can relieve the pain to some extent. Neuropathic pain can be treated by intercostal blockage since opioids in general have only a limited effect in this situation. The administration of anti epileptic drugs such as gabapentine or carbamazepine and anti depressive agents can also aid in pain treatment.

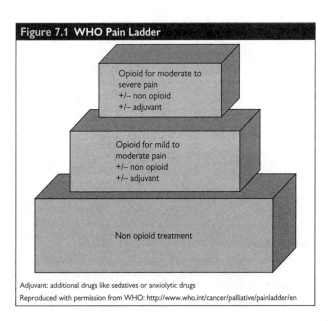

Figure 7.1 **WHO Pain Ladder**

Opioid for moderate to severe pain
+/– non opioid
+/– adjuvant

Opioid for mild to moderate pain
+/– non opioid
+/– adjuvant

Non opioid treatment

Adjuvant: additional drugs like sedatives or anxiolytic drugs

Reproduced with permission from WHO: http://www.who.int/cancer/palliative/painladder/en

7.2.2 Diffuse pain

The WHO guidelines for treatment of pain (Pain Ladder, Figure 7.1) can be used in the case of diffuse pain (Jadad & Browman, 1995). The first step is the administration of oral pain killers (e.g. paracetamol) with or without non steroidal anti-inflammatory drugs. The drugs should be given on a regular basis and if not effective the second step can include the use of moderately active opioids. This step can be omitted in most cancer patients and stronger opioids should be initiated without delay. In the case of nausea or swallowing difficulties the oral opioids should be replaced by trans-dermal patches.

7.3 Weight loss: anorexia and cachexia

The prevalence of weight loss in patients with lung cancer is 46%–61% and this is due to increased resting expenditure, related to the up-regulation of uncoupling proteins in skeletal muscle (Tisdale, 2009).

Anorexia is defined as the loss of appetite, combined with a decrease of food intake and is present in up to one-half of newly diagnosed cancer patients. It is characterized by caloric deficiency and increased fat metabolism.

Cachexia is the progressive weight loss associated with muscle wasting. It is believed that TNF-α, IL-6 and IFN-γ play a role in causing cachexia in cancer patients.

Unlike starvation, patients suffering from Cancer Cachexia Syndrome (CCS) lose both adipose and skeletal muscle mass, while preserving visceral muscle mass.

The clinical effects of cachexia include anorexia, weakness, fatigue, weight loss, muscle wasting, apathy, and impaired immuno-competence. In presence of cachexia, an increase in complications of surgery, radiotherapy and chemotherapy can be expected (Brown, 2002).

The therapeutic options for anorexia are dietary advice and nutritional supplementation and should be based on eating high calorie meals of small portions. In case of severe dysphagia because of radiation therapy a percutaneous endoscopic gastrostomy should be considered.

For cachexia, evidence based therapeutic options are missing. (Par)-enteral nutrition does not increase the survival and the symptomatic effects remain unclear. Also, some studies show that intensive nutrition in cachectic patients can lead up to 15% of morbidity due to the refeeding syndrome caused by a sudden shift from fat to carbohydrate metabolism and a sudden increase of insulin levels; resulting in an increased cellular uptake of phosphate. (Marinella, 2009).

The use of corticosteroids such as daily doses of prednisolone 40 mg (or dexamethasone 6 mg/day) leads to a short-lasting improvement for about 3–4 weeks, but the effects are subjective and are not accompanied by any improvement of the nutritional status. Prokinetic drugs such as metoclopramide 10–20 mg orally, 30 minutes before meals, or domperidone 10 mg are well tolerated in case of nausea.

Controlled trials have shown that progestational drugs such as medroxyprogesterone and megastrol acetate 480 mg/day may improve caloric intake and nutritional status because of the improvement of appetite and the sensation of wellbeing, but they may increase the risk of thromboenbolic events.

7.4 **Cough**

Tumours that are centrally located in the airways are more likely to cause cough. This is because of the location of cough receptors in the airways. In >65% of the patients cough is present at the time lung cancer is diagnosed. Persistent cough can cause headaches, insomnia, vomiting, rib fractures and syncope.

Symptomatic management of cough is guided by whether the cough produces sputum; the goal is either to promote expectoration of sputum or suppress the cough if it is non-productive (Joyce et al., 2008). Therapeutic options include the removal or reduction of the tumour by palliative radiation and/or chemotherapy. Endobronchial treatment options to relieve cough are seldom offered in absence of dyspnea or hemoptysis.

Medical treatment consists of centrally acting anti-tussives such as opioids and peripherally direct or indirect acting anti-tussives. For patients with cough and lung cancer the following centrally acting cough suppressant are recommended:

- Codeine 10–20 mg orally every 4–6 hours with a limit of 120 mg/ 24 hours
- Dihydrocodeine 10–30 mg orally three times a day with a daily dose no higher than 150 mg.
- Dextrometorphan 10–20 mg every 4–6 hours with the daily dose not to exceed 120 mg.

When the cancer itself causes the cough, bronchodilators and corticosteroids usually do not improve the symptoms.

Other cough management options are air humidification, the administration of nebulized mucolytic agents or opioids, and physiotherapy in order to promote expectoration of sputum.

7.5 **Dyspnea**

The prevalence of dyspnea in lung cancer patients varies from 55% to 87%. Many factors can contribute to dyspnea such as pleural effusion, pericardial effusion, severe anaemia, cachexia, and underlying COPD. Also, anxiety and depression may play an important role. Assessment of dyspnea may be challenging because of the subjective nature of the symptom. There are several tools to measure the 4 parameters: personal past history, variable mediators, patient's reactions to dyspnea, and outcomes of therapy. The visual analogue scale (VAS) is the easiest to use and is appropriate for repeated measurements of disease status.

Diagnostic testing includes pulse oximetry and full blood counts. In order to evaluate acute problems a chest radiograph is indicated. An important goal of assessment is to differentiate an acute cause of dyspnea from a condition that requires palliative interventions (Joyce et al., 2008).

In case of a short existing anaemia, Hb< 6 mmol/L, a transfusion with filtered erythrocytes is indicated. The initial treatment of symptomatic pleural effusions is the insertion of a chest tube and when possible followed by instillation of a sclerosing agent (chemical pleurodesis). In case of recurrent pleural effusion, prolonged pleural drainage with an indwelling catheter might be considered.

Oxygen therapy can relieve hypoxemic patients experiencing dyspnea. Routine use of oxygen for non-hypoxemic patients did not show benefit in clinical trials.

If dyspnea is the result of a central airway obstruction, radiation therapy (see below) or endobronchial intervention can improve this symptom.

There is strong evidence for the use of low dose opioids in patients with advanced disease experiencing dyspnea; morphine used to be the dominant opioid, but optimal dosage remains unclear. Fentanyl and furosemide are promising but need further confirmation. Treatment with albuterol and sustained-release theophylline seem to improve dyspnea in lung cancer patients with COPD.

7.6 **Fatigue**

Fatigue is a subjective sensation of exhaustion. Patients experiencing fatigue face psychological and physical problems due to a lack of energy. Fatigue in cancer patients has been associated with the dysregulation of the central serotonergic system and energy depletion of the muscle cells (Ahlberg et al.,).

In the early palliative phase it is necessary to determine symptoms like pain, dyspnea, itch, nausea. Iatrogenic symptoms and pharmacotherapy should be analysed and the additive effects of co-morbidity need to be clarified.

Clinical assessment for fatigue includes:

- Detection for anemia
- Physical appearance
- Shortness of breath
- Quality of sleep
- Pain
- Psychological issues.

Evidence for the symptomatic treatment of fatigue is limited, although some pharmaceutical options can be considered:

- Corticosteroids, e.g. prednisolone 20–40 mg/day
- Methylphenidate (Ritalin®) 10–20 mg, 2–3 times a day

Non-pharmaceutical options include:

- Balancing daily activities and rest
- Sleep hygiene practices such as sleeping at night and being awake during the day
- Exercise, e.g. walking.

7.7 Palliative radiotherapy

The primary goal of palliative radiotherapy is to ameliorate symptoms or to slow down the progression of the underlying tumour. Palliative radiotherapy can be considered for the following indications.

7.7.1 Dyspnea

When dyspnea is the result of endobronchial obstruction, short courses of radiation can be administered (see section on dyspnea). In general external radiation therapy is given but sometimes endobronchial radiation can be indicated, especially in case of previous radiotherapy and small, localized lesions. In the latter case Iridium 192 high dose irradiation is often used to deliver a local dose of 6–15 Gray at 1 cm distance of the catheter. This catheter is placed next to the tumour under fluoroscopic guidance using a bronchoscope. After securing the position, the iridium source is transported to the tumour site and remains there for 2–10 minutes.

7.7.2 Hemoptysis

During the course of lung cancer, endobronchial tumour localizations may bleed spontaneously, due to a bronchial infection or as a consequence of the previously administered therapy. This occurs in approximately 40% of the cases (Ripamont & Fusco, 2002). The patient may experience a short period of profuse bleeding or more chronic episodes with blood stained sputum. Radiotherapy in these cases is often successful. Depending on the location 1–3 fractions of 8 Gray can be administered.

7.7.3 Bone metastases

Painful lesions (bone metastases or direct growth of the tumour in the chest wall) are the most frequent indications for palliative radiotherapy. In 2/3 of the cases pain accompanies the lesion and in some cases there is an imminent risk of fracture. The metastases in the vertebral column are noteworthy for the high risk of spinal cord compression. These lesions are often good indications for radiation, especially when they are localized. In the majority of cases a single dose of 8 Gray is sufficient for optimal palliation and has been proven to be as effective as a more prolonged course of radiation with lower dose fractions (Konski et al., 2005). A significant effect on symptoms can be expected to occur within 3 weeks in 70–80% of the cases.

7.7.4 Brain metastases

Of all solid tumours, lung cancer has one of the highest incidences of brain metastases. Therapeutic interventions in this case depend on the general condition of the patient and life expectancy (Lagerwaard et al., 1999). In patients with good performance status there is a 60–90% chance of symptom control with whole brain radiation therapy.

7.7.5 Superior vena cava syndrome

This symptom can develop by local compression of the superior cava vein by the tumour or thrombosis of the vein, which are indicators for local radiation therapy. Using anticoagulant therapy in combination with the placement of an endovascular stent can be an alternative for this treatment.

7.8 Pleural effusions

During the course of many malignant diseases pleural fluid can develop. Usually a malignant pleural effusion presents unilaterally, it gives symptoms of cough and dyspnea, is blood tinged when tapped and contains malignant cells. When other causes are excluded (infectious, congestive heart failure, reactive), symptoms can be alleviated by a single pleural tap of 500–1500 ml. Thirty per cent of the responders to pleural tap can have a benefit for up to a few months after a single intervention, but most patients do require chest tube drainage with pleurodesis. In general patients are admitted for this procedure, which takes 3 to 7 days for complete evacuation and suction of the pleural effusion, followed by administration of a sclerosing agent (i.e. talc, tetracycline) and drain removal. In most publications a success rate of pleurodesis of 80% is reported but general surveys report a much lower rate of success (Burgers et al., 2008).

Currently out-patient treatments are tested using indwelling catheters and vacuum bottles that can be handled by the patient himself. This approach is also indicated in case of a so-called trapped lung where pleurodesis is not possible due to an incomplete expansion of the lung.

Pain

Goal: to optimize pain treatment
1. Identify underlying cause
2. Start oral pain meds early
3. Use Pain meds on a regular basis
4. The WHO pain ladder can be used with omission of the second step
5. Treat localized pain with radiation therapy
6. Trans-cutaneous and slow release opioids are often indicated.

Weight loss

Cause: loss of adipose and skeletal muscle tissue
Goal: to increase the general feeling of well being
1. Dietary advice: frequent meals of small portions with high calories (including use of supplements)
2. Consider percutaneous gastrostomy in case of swallowing problems
3. Corticosteroids result in a short lasting improvement (3–4 weeks) but also increase the general well being
4. Treat nausea optimally.

Cough

Cause: endobronchial lesions and/or infectious causes
1. In case of endobronchial lesions RT, surgery or local treatment is indicated
2. Symptomatic management can consist of codeine; dihydrocodeine or dextrometorphan (systemic or nebulized)
3. Treat infections accordingly.

Dyspnoea
Cause: obstruction of airways; oxygen diffusion
Limitation: treatment or patient related causes
1. Determine magnitude of dyspnoea and cause
2. Alleviate bronchial obstructions
3. Use bronchodilators when indicated
4. Correct anemia; congestive heart failure or pleural effusion
5. Oxygen therapy has limited effect
6. Treatment with sedation is indicated in advanced cases.

Further reading

Ahlberg K., Ekman T., Gaston-Johansson F., Mock V. Assessment and management of cancer-related fatigue in adults. *Lancet* **362**(9384): 640–50. Review.

Brown J.K. (2002) A systematic review of the evidence on symptom management of cancer-related anorexia and cachexia. *Oncol Nurs Forum* **29**(3): 517–32. Review.

Burgers J.A., Kunst P.W., Koolen M.G., Willems L.N., Burgers J.S., van den Heuvel M. (2008) Pleural drainage and pleurodesis: implementation of guidelines in four hospitals. *Eur Respir J* **32**(5): 1321–7.

Hollen P.J., Gralla R.J., Kris M.G., Potanovich L.M. (1993) Quality of life assessment in individuals with lung cancer: testing the Lung Cancer Symptom Scale (LCSS). *Eur J Cancer* **29A**(1): S51–8.

Jadad A.R., Browman G.P. (1995) The WHO analgesic ladder for cancer pain management. Stepping up the quality of its evaluation. *JAMA* **274**(23): 1870–3.

Joyce M., Schwartz S., Huhmann M. (2008) Supportive care in lung cancer. *Sem Oncol Nursing* **24**: 1:57–67.

Konski A., Feigenberg S., Chow E. (2005) Palliative radiation therapy. *Sem Oncol* **321**: 156–64.

Lagerwaard F.J., Levendag P.C., Nowak P.J.C.M., Eijkenboom W.M., Hanssens P.E., Schmitz P.I. (1999) Identification of prognostic factors in patients with brain metastases: a review of 1292 patients. *Int J Radiat Oncol Biol Phys* **43**: 795–803.

Marinella M.A. (2009) Refeeding syndrome: an important aspect of supportive oncology. *J Support Oncol* **7**(1): 11–6. Review.

Ripamont, C., Fusco F. (2002) Respiratory problems in advanced cancer. *Supp Care Cancer* **10**: 204–14.

Tisdale M.J. (2009) Mechanisms of cancer cachexia. *Physiol Rev* **89**(2): 381–410. Review.

Chapter 8

Development of new therapeutic agents for treatment of NSCLC

Arun Rajan and Giuseppe Giaccone

Key points

- Biologic therapies have become part of standard treatment of advanced NSCLC
- Novel biologic therapies are being developed for the treatment of NSCLC
- Targeting of ALK translocations has shown striking initial results in the treatment of tumors harboring ALK translocations/fusion events
- Clinical trials will have to be developed to evaluate the combination of cytotoxic chemotherapy and newer biologic therapies

8.1 Introduction

In recent years as more knowledge has been gained about the biology of lung cancer, newer targeted therapies have been developed, some of which are already being used for the treatment of patients with advanced disease. Many more biologic therapies are currently being evaluated in clinical trials. In this chapter we have outlined the major classes of biologic therapies in development for the treatment of NSCLC and highlighted important clinical trials evaluating these newer drugs.

8.2 Antiangiogenic therapy

The benefit of adding antiangiogenic therapy to standard chemotherapy is illustrated by the phase III ECOG study E4599 which compared the combination of bevacizumab with carboplatin and paclitaxel to carboplatin and paclitaxel alone. Significant improvements in progression free survival (PFS) and overall survival (OS) were seen in bevacizumab-treated patients (6.2 months v. 4.5 months, p<0.001; 12.3 months versus 10.3 months, p = 0.003) (Sandler *et al.*, 2006). Several phase II studies are currently ongoing that are evaluating the addition of bevacizumab to various platinum-based chemotherapy combinations in the first-line setting for patients with advanced NSCLC.

Other antiangiogenic strategies in the treatment of NSCLC involve the use of small molecule tyrosine kinase inhibitors (TKIs) directed against the vascular endothelial growth factor receptors (VEGFRs).

Cediranib (AZD2171) is an orally administered small molecule inhibitor of VEGFR-1, VEGFR-2, VEGFR-3, platelet-derived growth factor receptor beta (PDGFR-β), and c-kit. A phase II/III double-blind study with paclitaxel (200 mg/m^2) and carboplatin (AUC 6) administered every 3 weeks, with daily oral cediranib or placebo at 30 mg (first 45 patients received 45 mg) was recently reported (Goss *et al.*, 2010). The primary endpoint of the phase II part of the study was PFS with a plan to proceed with the phase III component of the study if the hazard ratio (HR) for PFS was $\leq$ 0.77 and the toxicity profile was acceptable. 296 patients were enrolled onto the study including 251 to the 30-mg cediranib cohort. An interim analysis of the phase II portion of the study (30-mg cohort) demonstrated a significantly higher response rate (RR) for cediranib than for placebo (38% v 16%; P $\leq$ .0001), and a HR of 0.77 for PFS (95% CI, 0.56 to 1.08). The study was halted to review imbalances in assigned causes of death between the two arms. Patients receiving cediranib had more hypertension, hypothyroidism, hand-foot syndrome, and GI toxicity. Among 296 patients assessed for survival 10 months after study unblinding, patients receiving cediranib had a slight survival benefit over those receiving placebo (median survival of 10.5 months v 10.1 months; HR, 0.78; 95% CI, 0.57 to 1.06; P = .11). Protocol-related toxicity accounted for significantly more deaths in the cediranib 30-mg cohort compared to no deaths due to protocol-related toxicity in the placebo group. Therefore, though the improved response and PFS with the addition of cediranib to carboplatin and paclitaxel in the first-line setting in patients with NSCLC appeared promising, the treatment did not appear to be well tolerated. Hence a randomized, double-blind, placebo-controlled trial of cediranib 20 mg with carboplatin and paclitaxel in advanced NSCLC has been initiated.

Vandetanib is an orally administered small molecule inhibitor of VEGFR-2, VEGFR-3, RET and EGFR that has shown modest activity as a single agent in patients with NSCLC (Kiura *et al.*, 2008). It has been evaluated in three large phase III trials in patients who progressed after first-line therapy. The ZEAL trial compared vandetanib plus pemetrexed to pemetrexed alone in the second-line setting in patients with advanced NSCLC with a primary objective of demonstrating an improvement in PFS. Vandetanib was administered orally at a dose of 100 mg/day with pemetrexed 500 mg/m^2 iv every 21 days for a maximum of 6 cycles. 534 patients were enrolled with a median age of 59 years, 21% had squamous histology, 256 patients received the combination of vandetanib plus pemetrexed and 278 patients received placebo plus pemetrexed. With a median duration of follow up of 9 months a trend towards improvement of PFS and OS was seen but this did not reach statistical significance (HR 0.86; CI 0.69 – 1.06; p = 0.108 and HR 0.86; CI 0.65 – 1.13; p = 0.219 respectively). However a statistically significant improvement in overall response rate was noted in the combination arm (19.1% v. 7.9%; p<0.001). The combination of vandetanib and pemetrexed was fairly well tolerated. Adverse effects were more frequent in the combination arm and included rash (38% v. 26%), diarrhea (26% v. 18%) and hypertension (12% v. 3%) (De Boer et al., 2009).

The ZODIAC trial evaluated the combination of vandetanib plus docetaxel versus docetaxel alone in patients who had failed first-line therapy. The primary endpoint was an improvement in PFS. Vandetanib 100 mg/day was administered orally with docetaxel 75 mg/m^2 every 21 days for a maximum of 6 cycles. 1391 patients were enrolled on this study with a mean age of 58 years, 25% patients had squamous histology, 694 patients received vandetanib plus docetaxel and 697 patients received placebo plus docetaxel. With a median follow up of 12.8 months the study met its primary objective of a statistically significant improvement in PFS for the combination arm (HR 0.79; CI 0.70 – 0.90; p<0.001). A significant improvement in overall response rate (17% v. 10%; p<0.001) and a trend towards improvement in overall survival was also seen (HR 0.91; CI 0.78 – 1.07; p=0.196). Common adverse effects in the combination arm were rash (42% v. 24%), diarrhoea (42% v. 33%), and neutropenia (32% v. 27%). This was the first phase III trial that demonstrated a significant improvement in clinical benefit when an oral targeted therapy was added to standard chemotherapy for treatment of advanced NSCLC (Herbst et al., 2009).

Vandetanib has also been evaluated against erlotinib in a randomized double-blind phase III trial after failure of first-line therapy (ZEST). Vandetanib was administered at a dose of 300 mg per day and erlotinib at a dose of 150 mg per day until progression or development of intolerable toxicity. The primary endpoint was an improvement in PFS. 1240 patients enrolled on the study with a mean age of 61 years. 22% patients had squamous histology, 623 patients received vandetanib and 617 patients received erlotinib. There was no improvement in PFS (HR 0.98; CI 0.87 – 1.10; p = 0.721), OS (HR 1.01; CI 0.89 – 1.16; p=0.830) or overall response rate (12% v. 12%). Adverse effects that were more common in the vandetanib arm included diarrhoea (50% v. 38%) and hypertension (16% v. 2%). A preplanned non-inferiority analysis for PFS and OS demonstrated equivalent efficacy for vandetanib and erlotinib (Natale *et al.*, 2009).

Given the contradictory results obtained in these three large phase III studies, the introduction of vandetanib in the treatment of advanced NSCLC appears uncertain.

Sorafenib is a multikinase inhibitor that targets the Ras/Raf/MEK/ERK signaling pathway VEGFRs 1, 2, and 3, PDGFR-β, fms-like tyrosine kinase receptor 3 (Flt-3), c-KIT and RET. In vitro studies have shown that sorafenib can deplete B-RAF, inhibit ERK phosphorylation, and induce G1 arrest in NSCLC cells with wild-type KRAS. However in cells with mutated KRAS, sorafenib depleted C-RAF and induced G1 arrest without affecting ERK phosphorylation (Takezawa *et al.*, 2009). Results from a phase II multicenter trial of sorafenib in patients with relapsed or refractory advanced NSCLC were reported recently (Blumenschein *et al.*, 2009). 52 patients received sorafenib at a dose of 400 mg orally twice a day; 51 patients were evaluable for efficacy. No objective responses were noted. However 30 patients (59%) achieved stable disease (SD). Median PFS was 2.7 months and median OS was 6.7 months. Major treatment related adverse events included skin toxicity in the form of hand-foot syndrome (10%), hypertension (4%), fatigue and diarrhoea (2% each). 1 patient experienced pulmonary haemorrhage that was thought to be drug-related. Although no objective responses were seen a significant proportion of patients experienced disease stabilization with an acceptable toxicity profile.

Two randomized phase III studies have been performed to evaluate sorafenib in combination with chemotherapy. The ESCAPE study randomized patients to receive carboplatin (AUC 6 on day 1), paclitaxel (200 mg/m^2 on day 1) and sorafenib or placebo (400 mg orally twice daily from day 2 to day 19) every 3 weeks. Daily sorafenib at a dose of 400 mg orally twice daily or placebo was continued as maintenance therapy after 6 cycles of chemotherapy. 926 patients were randomized and 464 patients received chemotherapy plus sorafenib. The median OS was 10.7 months in the group receiving sorafenib and 10.6 months in control arm (p = 0.93). Based on a planned interim analysis of efficacy the study was terminated for futility after 384 death events. Increased mortality was observed in patients with squamous histology randomized to the experimental arm (Scagliotti *et al.*, 2008). The NEXUS study was designed to evaluate the combination of cisplatin (75 mg/m^2 iv), gemcitabine (1250 mg/m^2 iv) and sorafenib (400 mg orally twice a day) against cisplatin, gemcitabine and placebo in the first-line therapy of patients with advanced NSCLC (NCT00449033). After the ESCAPE study was halted, the NEXUS study was amended to excluded patients with squamous histology. The results of this study are awaited. Recently a randomized phase III study has been initiated that compares sorafenib (400 mg orally twice daily) to placebo in patients with relapsed or refractory advanced predominantly non-squamous NSCLC after at least two but not more than three previous standard treatment regimens (NCT00863746).

Sunitinib malate (SU11248) is another oral, multikinase inhibitor of VEGFRs, PDGFRs, KIT, RET, and FLT3 that has demonstrated activity in NSCLC. In a phase II study 47 patients with recurrent advanced NSCLC were treated with sunitinib at a dose of 37.5 mg per day using a continuous dosing schedule. 1 PR (2%) and 8 SD (17%) lasting more than 3 months were seen. Median PFS was 12.1 wks (95% CI: 8.6–13.7). The most common treatment-related adverse events were fatigue/asthenia (15%), hypertension (6%), hypoxia (6%), dyspnea (4%), and hemoptysis (2%). One patient died due to possible treatment-related congestive heart failure (Brahmer et al., 2007). In another phase II study in patients with previously treated advanced NSCLC, sunitinib was administered at a dose of 50 mg per day on an intermittent schedule (4 weeks on and 2 weeks off). 63 patients were treated and 6 PRs (9.5%, 95% CI: 3.6–19.6%) and 12 SD (19.0%) were observed at the time of reporting. The most common grade 3/4 adverse events included fatigue/asthenia (21%), nausea (7%), vomiting (7%), abdominal pain (7%), and hypertension (5%). 3 patients died due to possible treatment-related complications: pulmonary haemorrhage (n = 2) and cerebral haemorrhage (n=1) (Socinski et al., 2006).

Axitinib (AG-013736) is an orally administered small molecule inhibitor of VEGFR-1, VEGFR-2, VEGFR-3, PDGFR-β and c-kit. It has been evaluated as a single-agent in a phase II study in patients with advanced NSCLC. 32 patients were enrolled and received axitinib at a starting dose of 5 mg orally twice daily. 9 out of 32 patients (28%) had received no prior chemotherapy for metastatic disease. 3 patients had a PR (9%) and 10 patients had SD (31%). Median duration of response was 8.3 months. Median PFS was 4.9 months in all patients and 9.2 months in those patients who had not received prior therapy for metastatic disease. Median OS was 14.8 months. The most common treatment-related adverse events were fatigue, anorexia, diarrhea and nausea. Grade 3 treatment-related adverse events seen in $\geq$ 5% of patients included fatigue (22%), hypertension (9%), and hyponatremia (9%) (Schiller et al., 2009). Axitinib is currently being evaluated in two phase II studies with cisplatin plus gemcitabine (for first-line treatment of squamous NSCLC; NCT00735904) and cisplatin plus pemetrexed for first-line treatment of non-squamous NSCLC; NCT00768755). A randomized phase II study of axitinib or bevacizumab in combination with paclitaxel and carboplatin as first line therapy for advanced NSCLC has also been conducted with a primary endpoint of PFS. (NCT00600821).

8.3 Anti-epidermal growth factor receptor (EGFR) therapy

The presence of sensitizing mutations in the EGFR genes confers sensitivity of NSCLC to EGFR tyrosine kinase inhibitors such as gefitinib and erlotinib. An analysis of clinical trials enrolling patients with NSCLC harbouring EGFR mutations and treated with EGFR TKIs in the first-line setting showed that the presence of sensitizing EGFR mutations was associated with a response rate of 67%, time to progression (TTP) of 11.8 months, and OS of 23.9 months. In contrast patients with wild-type EGFR treated with EGFR-TKIs in the first line setting had a response rate of 3% and TTP of 3.2 months (Jackman et al., 2009). Of the known mechanisms of de novo resistance to EGFR TKIs, the presence of K-Ras mutations in adenocarcinomas of the lung is probably the most common. Continued treatment of tumours harbouring EGFR sensitizing mutations with EGFR TKIs can lead to the development of acquired resistance. The most common mechanisms for the development of acquired resistance include the occurrence of a second resistant mutation such as the T790M, (accounting for ~50% of the cases), and c-Met amplification, (accounting for ~20% cases). Other less well-defined mechanisms of acquired resistance include presence of mutations in or activation of Her2/neu, or activation of other transmembrane receptors, such as IGF1R.

Irreversible small molecule inhibitors of the HER family of receptors are being evaluated in patients who develop acquired resistance to EGFR TKIs. PF-00299804 is an irreversible inhibitor of HER-1, HER-2, and HER-4 tyrosine kinases that is being evaluated in a phase II study in patients who have progressive disease after treatment with at least 1 line of chemotherapy and erlotinib. 66 patients with progressive NSCLC have been enrolled (44 adenocarcinoma; 22 non-adenocarcinoma) and received PF-00299804 at a dose of 45 mg orally once a day. Among the patients evaluable for response, 3 patients have had a confirmed PR. The clinical benefit rate (CR+PR+SD) beyond 6 weeks is 24 out of 36 (67%) in patients with adenocarcinoma and 2 out of 5 (40%) among non-adenocarcinomas. Prolonged stable disease has been seen in patients with T790M mutations and exon 20 insertions. Common adverse events include skin toxicity, diarrhea, fatigue, stomatitis, and emesis (Janne et al., 2009).

BIBW2992 is an irreversible dual inhibitor of EGFR and HER2 tyrosine kinases that is being evaluated in a phase II study in patients with adenocarcinoma of the lung and activating mutations of EGFR after failure of one line of chemotherapy (Shih et al., 2009). Out of 100 patients with tumours harbouring detectable EGFR mutations, 69 patients have started treatment with BIBW2992 at a dose of

50 mg orally once a day. Of 55 patients evaluable for response in the second line setting 29 (53%) have had a PR and 23 (42%) have had SD. The most common adverse events include diarrhoea (seen in 87% patients) and skin toxicity (seen in 88% patients).

An international phase II trial (LUX-Lung 2) evaluating BIBW2992 in NSCLC is currently underway. Patients with advanced NSCLC harboring activating mutations of EGFR exons 18 to 21 who have failed one line of cytotoxic chemotherapy are eligible. This trial also has a second stage for which chemotherapy-naïve patients meeting the above criteria will be eligible. The primary endpoint of LUX Lung 2 is determination of objective response rate. (NCT00525148).

LUX Lung 3 is a randomized phase III trial evaluating BIBW2992 against chemotherapy (cisplatin plus pemetrexed) as first line therapy for patients with advanced NSCLC harbouring activating mutations of EGFR with a primary endpoint of progression free survival. (NCT00949650).

BMS-690514 is an inhibitor of EGFR, HER2, and VEGFR1-3. In a phase I/II study patients with erlotinib-naïve and erlotinib-resistant advanced NSCLC were treated with BMS-690514 at a dose of 200 mg/d (Bahleda et al., 2009). Out of 60 patients treated, the disease control rate (CR+PR+SD lasting more than 4 months) was 11/28 (39%) among erlotinib-naïve patients and 7/32 (22%) among erlotinib-resistant patients. Tumour shrinkage was seen in one erlotinib-naïve patient harbouring a KRAS G13D mutation. Also two erlotinib-resistant patients with EGFR T790M mutations demonstrated SD. The most common treatment-related adverse events were diarrhoea (90%), skin rash (31%), asthenia (29%), anorexia (27%), hypertension (26%), and reversible acute renal insufficiency (11%). Currently a randomized phase II trial of BMS-690514 versus erlotinib in NSCLC is underway.

8.4 Targeting ALK translocations/fusion events

Translocations of the Anaplastic Lymphoma Kinase (ALK) gene located on chromosome 2p results in constitutive activation of ALK kinase and aberrant downstream signalling involving Akt, STAT3, and ERK1/2 (Amin, 2007). One of the fusion partners for the ALK gene is echinoderm microtubule-associated protein-like 4 (EML4). In a Japanese study EML4-ALK fusion has been reported in about 7% of NSCLC (Soda et al., 2007). Koivunen and colleagues screened 305 patients with NSCLC for the EML4-ALK fusion gene. 138 patients were from the US and 167 patients were from Korea. Four different variants of EML4-ALK fusion was detected in 8 of 305 cases (3%). All tumours harbouring the fusion gene were adenocarcinomas. Presence of the fusion gene was more commonly seen in never smokers or light smokers (< 10 pack-years) (6% vs. 1%; p=0.049). No tumours had concurrent KRAS or BRAF mutations; however one tumour harboured a concurrent EGFR kinase mutation (del E746_A750) (Koivunen et al., 2008). Shaw and colleagues presented data from a large series of 141 patients with NSCLC screened for the EML4-ALK fusion gene. 18 patients (13%) harboured the ALK translocation and 31 patients (22%) were EGFR mutant. Patients with the ALK translocation were younger (median age 52.5 years vs. 64 years; p = 0.003), more likely to be male (61% vs. 30%; p = 0.015), and more likely to be light or never smokers (100% vs. 43%; p<0.001) (Shaw et al., 2009). Data from a phase 1 dose-escalation trial of PF-02341066, a selective small molecule inhibitor of c-MET/HGFR and ALK receptor tyrosine kinases showed that out of 10 patients with NSCLC harbouring the EML4-ALK rearrangement, 1 patient had a PR, 2 patients had an unconfirmed PR and 4 patients had SD (Kwak et al., 2009). Hence treatment directed against the EML4-ALK fusion product has demonstrated promising clinical activity in the subset of patients with tumours harbouring ALK translocations. PF-02341066 is currently being evaluated in a phase III clinical trial in patients with NSCLC harboring the EML4-ALK translocation who have failed at least one previous platinum-containing chemotherapy regimen. (NCT00932893). Patients are randomized to receive PF-02341066 at a dose of 250 mg orally twice a day using a continuous schedule or either pemetrexed 500 mg/m^2 iv on day 1 of a 21-day cycle or docetaxel 75 mg/m^2 iv on day 1 of a 21-day cycle.

8.5 Targeting RAS mutations in NSCLC

The product of RAS genes consist of a family of GTP-binding proteins that regulate cell growth, differentiation, and apoptosis. Downstream effectors include the MAPK, STAT and PI3K signalling pathways. 10% to 15% of NSCLCs harbour RAS mutations the vast majority of which are KRAS mutations (Vojtek & Der, 1998; Riley et al., 2009). Tumours harbouring RAS mutations demonstrate primary resistance to EGFR TKIs such as erlotinib.

Farnesylthiosalicylic acid (salirasib) is being evaluated for the treatment of RAS mutants. Preliminary results of a phase II trial of salirasib in patients with advanced adenocarcinoma of the lung enriched for KRAS mutations showed no objective responses. However 8 out of 26 patients showed stable disease (28% in previously treated patients with KRAS mutations and 38% in previously untreated patients) and the median time to progression in these two groups was 1 month and 2 months respectively (Johnson et al., 2009).

8.6 **Mitogen-activated protein kinase kinase (MEK) 1/2 inhibitor**

MEK is a component of the mitogen activated protein (MAP) kinase pathway that is present downstream of EGFR. AZD6244 is a potent inhibitor of MEK that has been evaluated in a two-part phase I study in patients with advanced cancers. 57 patients were enrolled and the MTD was determined to be 200 mg orally twice a day. However this dose was found to be poorly tolerated and patients were treated at a dose of 100 mg orally twice a day. The most common grade 3/4 adverse effect was development of a rash. RAF and RAS mutations were detected in 10 out of 26 assessable tumour samples. 9 patients had stable disease for at least 5 months (Adjei *et al.*, 2008). AZD6244 (100 mg PO BID) has also been evaluated against pemetrexed (500 mg/m^2 iv every 3 weeks) in a randomized phase II study in the second and third-line treatment of patients with NSCLC. 84 patients enrolled and 40 were randomized to receive AZD6244. 2 responses were seen in each arm (RR: 5% for AZD6244 and 4.5% for pemetrexed). Disease progression was seen in 28 patients (70%) in the AZD6244 arm and 26 patients (59%) in the pemetrexed arm (HR 1.35; 80% CI 0.93–1.54; p = 0.30). Median PFS in the two arms was 67 days and 90 days respectively (HR 1.08; 80% CI 0.75 – 1.54; p = 0.79). The most common adverse events in the AZD6244 arm were skin rash (43%), diarrhoea (33%), nausea, and vomiting (20% each) Tzekova *et al.*, 2008). In an ongoing double-blind, randomized phase II study, the combination of AZD6244 (75 mg orally twice daily) and docetaxel (75 mg/m^2 every 21 days) is being evaluated against docetaxel alone in KRAS mutation positive NSCLC with PFS as the primary endpoint.

8.7 **Heat shock protein inhibition in NSCLC**

A study using genome-wide screening to detect chromosomal copy number changes in patients with radically resected stage I and II NSCLC, showed a deletion in chromosome 14q in 44% cases. This deletion influenced gene expression for Hsp90 and correlated with better overall survival (p = 0.008) (Gallegos Ruiz *et al.*, 2008). Further evidence of the contribution of Hsp90 in the pathogenesis of lung cancer comes from a study by Sos *et al.* who show that the presence of KRAS mutations in a panel of NSCLC cell lines is associated with Hsp90 dependency. The authors also showed that mice with adenocarcinoma harbouring KRAS mutations had significant tumour shrinkage when treated with an Hsp90 inhibitor (Sos *et al.*, 2009).

IPI-504 is an Hsp90 inhibitor that causes degradation of mutated EGFR and cMET in NSCLC cell lines. Results from a phase II study of

IPI-504 in patients with relapsed or refractory advanced NSCLC were reported at ASCO 2009. 43 patients had been enrolled of which 10 patients had mutated EGFR and 17 patients had no EGFR mutations. In 24 evaluable patients (11 with no EGFR mutations; 8 with EGFR mutations), 2 PRs and 8 SD lasting more than 12 weeks were noted. Interestingly both PRs and 7 out of 8 patients with SD had wild-type EGFR. Treatment with IPI-504 was well tolerated and common adverse events included fatigue, nausea, and diarrhoea (Sequist et al., 2009).

8.8 Insulin-like growth factor receptor antagonists

The Insulin-Like Growth Factor (IGF) system is involved in signal transduction from the cell surface to the ERK/MEK and phosphatidylinositol 3-kinase (PI3K)/Akt pathways. Aberrant functioning of the IGF system has been associated with a higher incidence and severity of lung cancer (Spitz et al., 2002). Figitumumab (CP-751871) is a highly potent IGF-1R antibody that has been evaluated in patients with NSCLC. In a randomized phase II study the combination of figitumumab (10 mg/kg or 20 mg/kg), carboplatin (AUC 6) and paclitaxel (200 mg/m^2) versus carboplatin and paclitaxel alone was evaluated in the first-line setting in NSCLC. 43 of 85 patients (51%) receiving the three drug combination had objective responses compared to 21 of 58 patients (36%; p<0.001) receiving chemotherapy alone. Among the patients with squamous cell carcinoma histology, 13 of 18 (72%) patients responded to the three drug combination as compared to 5 of 12 patients (42%; p<0.001) who responded to chemotherapy alone (Karp et al., 2008). A single arm trial extension cohort was conducted to confirm activity in patients with squamous cell histology. 56 patients with non-adenocarcinoma NSCLC were enrolled and received paclitaxel (200 mg/m^2), carboplatin (AUC of 6) and figitumumab (20 mg/kg) every three weeks for up to 6 cycles. Patients who had a response or stable disease were eligible to continue treatment with figitumumab as a single agent until disease progression. Among patients with squamous cell carcinoma, 25 out of 40 patients responded including 1 complete response. Median progression free survival had not been reached after 4 months follow up (Karp et al., 2009). A large phase III study of CP-751,871 in combination with paclitaxel and carboplatin versus paclitaxel and carboplatin in patients with predominantly squamous cell, large cell or adenosquamous NSCLC was launched in March 2008 (NCT00596830). However the study was halted in September 2009 when an increased number of serious adverse effects including fatalities were noted in the experimental arm. The study had accrued

681 patients out of 820 patients when accrual was stopped. In December 2009 this study was discontinued for futility when an analysis by an independent Data Safety Monitoring Committee (DSMC) showed that the addition of CP-751871 to paclitaxel plus carboplatin would be unlikely to meet the primary endpoint of improving overall survival compared to paclitaxel plus carboplatin alone.

Other studies that are evaluating IGF-1R inhibitors in NSCLC include a phase I dose-escalation study of CP-751871 in combination with cisplatin and gemcitabine in previously untreated patients with advanced NSCLC (NCT00560573). The study was amended in September 2008 to evaluate the combination of CP-751871 in combination with cisplatin and pemetrexed in previously untreated patients with NSCLC. The treatment plan consists of CP-751871 administered at doses ranging from 6 mg/kg to 20 mg/kg on day 1 in combination with cisplatin 75 mg/m^2 plus pemetrexed 500 mg/m^2 administered on day 1 of a 21-day cycle up to 6 cycles, or cisplatin 80 mg/m^2 on day 1 in combination with gemcitabine 1250 mg/m^2 on days 1 and 8 of a 21-day cycle up to 6 cycles.

The IGF-1R inhibitor IMC-A12 is being evaluated in a phase II cross over study with a safety lead in in combination with erlotinib compared with erlotinib alone in patients with advanced NSLC who have failed at least one platinum-containing chemotherapy regimen. IMC-A12 is administered on days 1, 8, 15, and 22 of a 28 day cycle and erlotinib is administered once daily on days 1–28 (NCT00778167).

8.9 Histone deacetylase inhibitors

Transcriptional activity of a number of genes is determined by the degree of histone acetylation, which in turn is a function of the relative activity of histone acetyltransferase and histone deacetylase. Histone deacetylase (HDAC) inhibitors can activate apoptotic pathways and caused cell death (Peart et al., 2005). In addition, the effect of HDAC inhibitors on non-histone proteins such as Hsp90 and tubulin is also responsible for their anticancer activity. Overexpression of HDACs in NSCLC provides the therapeutic basis for the use of HDAC inhibitors either as single-agents or as a component of combination therapy for NSCLC (Sasaki et al., 2004).

Vorinostat (suberoylanilide hydroxamic acid/SAHA) is a small molecule inhibitor of HDAC. Preclinical studies have demonstrated the antiproliferative and pro-apoptotic activity of Vorinostat on NSCLC cell lines (Miyanaga et al., 2008). In a phase I study the combination of vorinostat, carboplatin and paclitaxel was evaluated in advanced solid malignancies. Vorinostat was used at a dose of

400 mg orally once a day for 14 days or 300 mg orally twice daily for 7 days along with carboplatin (AUC6) and paclitaxel (200 mg/m^2). 25 patients were evaluable for response; 11 PRs and 7 SD were seen. Of 19 patients with NSCLC (18 patients were chemotherapy-naïve) enrolled on this study, 10 PRs and 4 SD were seen. Toxicities associated with treatment included febrile neutropenia (2 patients on the 400 mg QD schedule), grade 3/4 non-febrile neutropenia (22 patients), grade 3/4 thrombocytopenia (11 patients), nausea, emesis, diarrhoea, anemia, fatigue, and neuropathy (Ramalingam et al., 2007). The combination of Vorinostat (400 mg orally once daily), carboplatin (AUC6) and paclitaxel (200 mg/m^2) was evaluated in a phase II/III study with a primary endpoint of improvement in overall survival (NCT00473889). However this study was terminated based on the results of a pre-planned interim analysis that showed that the primary endpoint had not been achieved. Further, the same combination (with similar doses of the three drugs and Vorinostat given for 14 days out of 21 days and chemotherapy repeated every 3 weeks) has been evaluated in a randomized, double-blinded, placebo-controlled phase II study with a primary endpoint of response rate (NCT00481078). 94 patients were enrolled. The response rate in the Vorinostat arm was 34% versus 12.5% in the placebo arm (p = 0.02). Median PFS and OS in the Vorinostat arm was 6 months (versus 4.1 months; p=0.48) and 13 months (versus 9.7 months; p = 0.17) (Ramalingam et al., 2010). A phase II study of single-agent vorinostat at a dose of 400 mg orally once daily, was conducted in patients with relapsed NSCLC. 16 patients were enrolled on this study of which 14 patients were evaluable for response. No objective responses were noted. However 8 patients had SD, median TTP was 2.3 months, and median OS was 7.2 months. Significant adverse effects possibly related to treatment included acute ischemic stroke, neutropenia, lymphopenia, fatigue, dehydration, venous thromboembolism (PE/DVT) (Traynor et al., 2009).

8.10 **Modulators of apoptosis**

Apoptosis (programmed cell death) can be triggered by a number of factors that act through a family of cysteine proteases known as caspases. The extrinsic apoptotic pathway is activated by the binding of ligands to specific cell surface receptors (death receptors). Tumour necrosis factor-related apoptosis-inducing ligand (TRAIL) binds to its specific receptors TRAIL receptor 1 and TRAIL receptor 2 and induces apoptosis.

Mapatumumab is a fully human monoclonal antibody that targets TRAIL receptor 1. A phase 1 study evaluated the combination of mapatumumab with gemcitabine and cisplatin in patients with advanced solid tumours. 49 patients (including 3 patients with NSCLC) were treated with gemcitabine 1250 mg/m^2 intravenously (i.v.) on days 1 and 8, cisplatin 80 mg/m2 i.v. on day 1, and mapatumumab administered i.v. in escalating doses as part of a 21-day cycle. 12 PRs and 25 SD were seen. The combination was well tolerated at doses up to 30 mg/kg (Mom et al., 2009). Mapatumumab has also been evaluated in combination with carboplatin and paclitaxel in a phase I study. 27 patients with advanced solid malignancies (including 6 patients with NSCLC and 1 patient with small-cell lung cancer) received mapatumumab at doses of 3 mg/kg, 10 mg/kg or 20 mg/kg along with carboplatin (AUC6) and paclitaxel (200 mg/m^2) every 21 days for up to 6 cycles. 5 patients achieved PR (including 2 NSCLC) and 12 patients had SD as best response. Mapatumumab was well tolerated at doses up to 20 mg/kg along with carboplatin and paclitaxel (Leong et al., 2009). In a randomized phase II trial, the combination of carboplatin, paclitaxel and mapatumumab is being evaluated as first line therapy in NSCLC with primary outcome measures of objective response and PFS. (NCT00583830).

AMG 951 [rhApo2L/TRAIL] is a dual pro-apoptotic receptor agonist that is being evaluated with carboplatin, paclitaxel with or without bevacizumab in a randomized phase II trial for first-line treatment of NSCLC. The primary end point of the study is determination of the objective response rate. (NCT00508625).

Survivin is an antiapoptotic protein that inhibits caspase activation. Increased expression of survivin is seen in many tumour types including NSCLC, and an inverse correlation has been noted between increased expression of survivin and prognosis (Giaccone et al., 2009).

YM155 is a small molecule inhibitor of survivin gene expression that reduces survivin protein levels and specifically inhibits survivin-mediated apoptosis while not affecting other apoptotic pathways. A phase II study was conducted to evaluate the antitumour activity of YM155 in patients with advanced NSCLC who had received at least one prior platinum-based chemotherapy regimen. Patients were treated with YM155 at a dose of 4.8 mg/m^2/day administered as a continuous i.v. infusion over 168 hours as part of a 21-day cycle. 37 patients were treated and 2 PRs (5.4%) and 14 SD (37.8%) were noted. Median PFS was 1.7 months, median OS was 6.6 months, and 1-year survival was 35.1%. Treatment was well tolerated and the most common treatment-related adverse events included fatigue (27%), pyrexia (16%), chills (11%), and nausea (11%). [42]

8.11 **Conclusions**

Management of advanced lung cancer continues to remain a challenging prospect. As more insight is gained into the biology of the disease, it has spurred the development of newer biologic therapies that are in various phases of development. With the exception of rare mutational events, it seems less likely that a single targeted drug will be able to adequately treat most patients with advanced NSCLC. Hence future effects should be directed towards the combination of novel targeted therapies with currently available cytotoxic chemotherapy or other targeted agents.

References

Adjei A.A., Cohen R.B., Franklin W., et al. (2008) Phase I Pharmacokinetic and pharmacodynamic study of the oral, small-molecule mitogen-activated protein kinase kinase 1/2 inhibitor AZD6244 (ARRY-142886) in patients with advanced cancer. *J Clin Oncol* **26**: 2139–46.

Amin H.M., Lai R. (2007) Pathobiology of ALK+ Anaplastic large-cell lymphoma. *Blood* **110**: 2259–67.

Bahleda R., Soria J., Harbison C., et al. (2009) Tumor regression and pharmacodynamic (PD) biomarker validation in non-small cell lung cancer (NSCLC) patients treated with the ErbB/VEGFR inhibitor BMS-690514. *J Clin Oncol* **27**(15s): abstract 8098.

Blumenschein Jr G.R., Gatzemeier U., Fossella F., et al. (2009) Phase II, multicenter, uncontrolled trial of single-agent sorafenib in patients with relapsed or refractory, advanced non-small-cell lung cancer. *J Clin Oncol* **27**: 4274–80.

Brahmer J.R., Govindan R., Novello S., et al. (2007) Efficacy and safety of continuous daily sunitinib dosing in previously treated advanced non-small cell lung cancer (NSCLC). Results from a phase II study. *J Clin Oncol* **25**(18S): abstract 7542.

De Boer R., Arrieta O., Gottfried M., et al. (2009) Vandetanib plus pemetrexed versus pemetrexed as second-line therapy in patients with advanced non-small cell lung cancer (NSCLC): A randomized, double-blind phase III trial (ZEAL). *J Clin Oncol* **27**(15s): abstract 8010.

Gallegos Ruiz M.I., Floor K., Roepman P., et al. (2008) Integration of gene dosage and gene expression in mom-small cell lung cancer, identification of HSP90 as potential target. *PLoS ONE* **3**(3): e0001722.

Giaccone G., Zatloukal P., Roubec J., et al. (2009) Multicenter phase II trial of YM155, a small-molecule suppressor of survivin, in patients with advanced, refractory, non-small-cell lung cancer. *J Clin Oncol* **27**: 4481–86.

Goss G.D., Arnold A., Shepherd F.A., et al. (2010) Randomized, double-blind trial of carboplatin and paclitaxel with either daily oral cediranib or placebo in advanced non–small-cell lung cancer: NCIC Clinical Trials Group BR24 Study. *J Clin Oncol* **28**: 49–55.

Herbst R.S., Sun Y., Korfee S., *et al.* (2009) Vandetanib plus docetaxel versus docetaxel as second-line treatment for patients with advanced non-small cell lung cancer (NSCLC): A randomized, double-blind phase III trial (ZODIAC). *J Clin Oncol* **27**(18s): abstract CRA8003.

Jackman D.M., Miller V.A., Cioffredi L.A., *et al* (2009). Impact of epidermal growth factor receptor and KRAS mutations on clinical outcomes in previously untreated non-small cell lung cancer patients: results of an online tumor registry of clinical trials. *Clin Cancer Res* **15**: 5267–73.

Janne P.A., Reckamp K., Koczywas M., *et al.* (2009) A Phase 2 Trial of PF-00299804 (PF299), an oral irreversible HER tyrosine kinase inhibitor (TKI), in patients (pts) with advanced NSCLC after failure of prior chemotherapy and erlotinib: preliminary efficacy and safety results. 13th World Conference on Lung Cancer, San Francisco 2–6 September 2009, suppl. *J Thor Oncol*: Abstract a31.

Johnson M.L., Rizvi N.A., Ginsberg M.S., *et al.* (2009) A phase II trial of salirasib in patients with stage III/IV lung adenocarcinoma enriched for KRAS mutations. *J Clin Oncol* **27**(15s): abstract 8012.

Karp D.D., Novello S., Cardenal F., *et al.* (2009) Continued high activity of figitumumab (CP-751,871) combination therapy in squamous lung cancer. *J Clin Oncol* **27**(15s): abstract 8072.

Karp D.D., Paz-Ares L.G., Novello S., *et al.* (2008) High activity of the anti-IGF-1R antibody CP-751,871 in combination with paclitaxel and carboplatin in squamous NSCLC. *J Clin Oncol* **26**(15s): abstract 8015.

Kiura K., Nakagawa K., Shinkai T., *et al.* (2008) A randomized, double-blind, phase IIa dose-finding study of Vandetanib (ZD6474) in Japanese patients with non-small cell lung cancer. *J Thorac Oncol* **3**: 386–93.

Koivunen J.P., Mermel C., Zejnullahu K., *et al.* (2008) EML4-ALK fusion gene and efficacy of an ALK kinase inhibitor in lung cancer. *Clin Cancer Res* **14**: 4275–83.

Kwak E.L., Camidge D.R., Clark J., *et al.* (2009) Clinical activity observed in a phase I dose escalation trial of an oral c-met and ALK inhibitor, PF-02341066. *J Clin Oncol* **27**(15s): abstract 3509.

Leong S., Cohen R.B., Gustafson D.L., *et al.* (2009) Mapatumumab, an antibody targeting TRAIL-R1, in combination with paclitaxel and carboplatin in patients with advanced solid malignancies: results of a phase I and pharmacokinetic study. *J Clin Oncol* **27**: 4413–21.

Miyanaga A., Gemma A., Noro R., *et al.* (2008) Antitumor activity of histone deacetylase inhibitors in non-small cell lung cancer cells: development of a molecular predictive model. *Mol Cancer Ther* **7**: 1923–30.

Mom C.H., Verweij J., Oldenhuis C.N., *et al.* (2009) Mapatumumab, a fully human agonistic monoclonal antibody that targets TRAIL-R1, in combination with gemcitabine and cisplatin: a phase I study. *Clin Cancer Res* **15**: 5584–90.

Monzo M., Rosell R., Felip E., *et al.* (1999) A novel anti-apoptosis gene: Re-expression of survivin messenger RNA as a prognosis marker in non-small-cell lung cancers. *J Clin Oncol* **17**: 2100–04.

Natale R.B., Thongprasert S., Greco F.A., *et al.* (2009) Vandetanib versus erlotinib in patients with advanced non-small cell lung cancer (NSCLC) after failure of at least one prior cytotoxic chemotherapy: A randomized, double-blind phase III trial (ZEST). *J Clin Oncol* **27**(15s): abstract 8009.

Peart M.J., Smyth G.K., van Laar R.K., *et al.* (2005) Identification and functional significance of genes regulated by structurally different histone deacetylase inhibitors. *Proc Natl Acad Sci USA* **102**: 3697–3702.

Ramalingam S.S., Maitland M.L., Frankel P., *et al.* (2010) Carboplatin and paclitaxel in combination with either vorinostat or placebo for first-line therapy of advanced non-small cell lung cancer. *J Clin Oncol* **28**: 56–62.

Ramalingam S.S., Parise R.A., Ramanathan R.K., *et al.* (2007) Phase I and pharmacokinetic study of vorinostat, a histone deacetylase inhibitor, in combination with carboplatin and paclitaxel for advanced solid malignancies. *Clin Cancer Res* **13**: 3605–10.

Riley G.J., Marks J., Pao W. (2009) K-RAS mutations in non-small cell lung cancer *Proc Am Thorac Soc* **6**: 201–5.

Sandler A., Gray R., Perry M.C., *et al.* (2006) Paclitaxel-carboplatin alone or with bevacizumab for non-small cell lung cancer. *N Engl J Med* **355**: 2542–50.

Sasaki H., Moriyama S., Nakashima Y., *et al.* (2004) Histone deacetylase 1 mRNA expression in lung cancer. *Lung Cancer* **46**: 171–8.

Scagliotti G., von Pawel J., Reck M., *et al.* (2008) Sorafenib plus carboplatin/paclitaxel in chemonaive patients with stage IIIB-IV non-small cell lung cancer (NSCLC): Interim analysis (IA) results from the phase III, randomized, double-blind, placebo-controlled, ESCAPE (Evaluation of Sorafenib, Carboplatin And Palitaxel Efficacy in NSCLC) trial. *J Thorac Oncol* **3**(1): S97(abstract 275O).

Sequist L.V., Gettinger S., Natale R., *et al.* (2009) A phase II trial of IPI-504 (retaspimycin hydrochloride), a novel Hsp90 inhibitor, in patients with relapsed and/or refractory stage IIIb or stage IV non-small cell lung cancer (NSCLC) stratified by EGFR mutation status. *J Clin Oncol* **27**(15s): abstract 8073.

Shaw A.T., Costa D., Mino-Kenudson M., *et al.* (2009) Clinicopathologic features of EML4-ALK mutant lung cancer. *J Clin Oncol* **27**(15s): abstract 11021.

Shih J., Yang C., Su W., *et al.* (2009) A phase II study of BIBW2992, a novel irreversible dual EGFR and HER2 tyrosine kinase inhibitor (TKI), in patients with adenocarcinoma of the lung and activating EGFR mutations after failure of one line of chemotherapy (LUX-Lung 2) *J Clin Oncol* **27**(15s): abstract 8013.

Schiller J.H., Larson T., Ou S.H., *et al.* (2009) Efficacy and safety of axitnib in patients with advanced non-small-cell lung cancer: results from a phase II study. *J Clin Oncol* **27**: 3836–41.

Socinski M.A., Novello S., Sanchez J.M. *et al.* (2006) Efficacy and safety of sunitinib in previously treated, advanced non-small cell lung cancer (NSCLC): Preliminary results of a multicenter phase II trial. *J Clin Oncol* **24**(18S): abstract 7001.

Soda M., Choi Y.L., Enomoto M., *et al.* (2007) Identification of the transforming EML4-ALK fusion gene in non-small-cell lung cancer. *Nature* **448**: 561–6.

Sos M.L., Michel K., Zander T., *et al.* (2009) Predicting drug susceptibility of non-small cell lung cancers based on genetic lesions. *J Clin Invest* **119**: 1727–40.

Spitz M.R., Barnett M.J., Goodman G.E., *et al.* (2002) Serum insulin like growth factor (IGF) and IGF binding protein levels and risk of lung cancer: a case control study nested in the beta carotene and retinol efficacy trial cohort. *Cancer Epidemiol Biomarkers Prev* **11**: 1413–8.

Takezawa K., Okamoto I., Yonesaka K., *et al.* (2009) Sorafenib inhibits non-small cell lung cancer cell growth by targeting B-RAF in KRAS wild-type cells and C-RAF in KRAS mutant cells (2009). *Cancer Res* **69**(16): 6515–21.

Traynor A.M., Dubey S., Eickhoff J.C., *et al.* (2009) Vorinostat (NSC# 701852) in patients with relapsed non-small cell lung cancer. *J Thorac Oncol* **4**: 522–6.

Tzekova V., Cebotaru C., Ciuleanu T.E., *et al.* (2008) Efficacy and safety of AZD6244 (ARRY-142886) as second/third-line treatment of patients with advanced non-small cell lung cancer. *J Clin Oncol* **26** (May 20 suppl.): abstract 8029.

Vojtek A., Der C. (1998) Increasing complexity of the ras signaling pathway. *J Biol Chem* **273**:19925–8.

Index

111